Nematodes - From the Past to the Future

Edited by Nihal Dogan

Published in London, United Kingdom

Nematodes - From the Past to the Future
http://dx.doi.org/10.5772/intechopen.1008035
Edited by Nihal Dogan

Contributors
Chunda Feng, John E. Erpelding, Mukesh R. Siddhapara, Nchore Shem Bonuke, Nihal Dogan, Salliana R. Stetina, Sonam Kumari, Thattankandy Meethal Aparna, Tinatin Doolotkeldieva, Waceke Joyce Wajohi, Waswa Stanlous Juma

First published in London, United Kingdom, 2026 by IntechOpen
IntechOpen is the global imprint of INTECHOPEN LIMITED, registered in England and Wales, registration number: 11086078, 167-169 Great Portland Street, London, W1W 5PF, United Kingdom

For EU product safety concerns: IN TECH d.o.o., Prolaz Marije Krucifikse Kozulić 3, 51000 Rijeka, Croatia, info@intechopen.com or visit our website at intechopen.com.

British Library Cataloguing-in-Publication Data
A catalogue record for this book is available from the British Library

Nematodes - From the Past to the Future
Edited by Nihal Dogan
p. cm.
Print ISBN 978-1-83634-677-7
Online ISBN 978-1-83634-676-0
eBook (PDF) ISBN 978-1-83634-678-4

Meet the editor

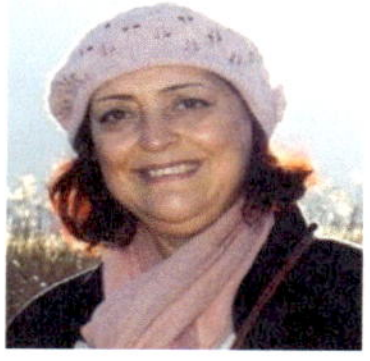

Prof. Dr. Nihal Dogan has worked in the Department of Microbiology, Faculty of Medicine, Osmangazi University, Turkey, since 1986. Her master's and Ph.D. theses focused on the diagnosis and sero-epidemiology of toxoplasmosis. She was a visiting researcher on the diagnosis of Entamoeba histolytica at the University of Virginia, USA, in 2003, and an observer researcher working on trypanosomes at the Faculty of Medicine, Universidad De Chile, in 2016. She was appointed a professor in 2008 and is the leading academic in the field of parasitology, with expertise in the epidemiology of parasitic diseases. Her research interests include medical ethics, seroepidemiological surveys, intestinal, blood, tissue, and ocular parasites, vector-borne diseases, and zoonotic parasites. Her research has been published in more than 40 national and international journals. She also made 85 poster presentations, as well as numerous oral presentations and keynote speeches, at international and national congresses. She has written numerous book chapters on infectious diseases, clinical parasitology, and clinical microbiology, as well as medical microbiology laboratory applications and manuals.

Contents

Preface

The phylum *Nematoda*, commonly known as nematodes or roundworms, represents a very large group within the animal kingdom. As phylogenetic studies continue, new species are being added to the systematic classification. A 2013 animal biodiversity study reported over 25,000 species, while DNA barcoding studies estimate the existence of approximately 1 million species. Their ability to adapt easily to any ecosystem plays a major role in their enormous diversity. Thus, some species can inhabit any part of the Earth's lithosphere, ranging from the Arctic region to the tropical belt. Nematodes represent 90% of the animals on the ocean floor, where the number of living organisms is relatively low. At the same time, they also constitute a significant portion of the animal population on the soil surface. It is estimated that about one-third of them are parasites in humans and other vertebrates.

Their classification was initiated in 1758 by Carl Linnaeus as *Ascaris* and *Dracunculus*, two important nematode species affecting human health. Their systematics have undergone continuous changes up to the present day. In 2022, based on molecular and morphological evidence, they were divided into the classes *Enoplea, Dorylaimida, Chromadorea*, and numerous subclasses belonging to them.

A significant number of members of this group, in addition to species that parasitize humans and many animal species, can cause significant economic losses in plants. A significant proportion of nematodes affecting human health worldwide are soil-borne species. These are called soil-transmitted nematodes and are among the leading causes of high mortality and morbidity from parasitic infections associated with developmental delays in children, especially in developing countries. In addition to soil-borne nematodes such as Ascaris, hookworms, whipworms, Trichinella, and Baylisascaris, vector-borne filarial nematodes are also among the most common causative agents to notice. Among those commonly seen in humans, their sizes range from microscopic to 1 meter in length. The mouth, located in the cylindrical head section, has 3-6 lip structures. The mouth contains cutting plates resembling teeth. The outer surface of the body is covered by 2-3 layers of cuticle resembling epidermis. Almost all are dioecious, with females laying eggs that are either embryonated or non-embryonated.

A significant number of nematodes live freely in soil and water and feed on various microorganisms. Their sizes vary considerably, and their bodies are cylindrical with pointed ends. Paleontological studies have shown that they are among the oldest parasites of humans. In addition to affecting animal health and causing significant losses in livestock farming, nematodes also cause important zoonotic infections.

While some nematodes provide significant benefits for plant health, others attack plants, sucking their sap, carrying various harmful organisms, and causing damage by acting as vectors. However, it is important to remember that some species can be used in biological control as an alternative to pesticides that negatively affect human and animal health. For example, they play an important role in the soil nitrogen cycle, as well as regulating soil bacterial colonization by feeding on them. Commensalism is one of the most common relationships between nematodes and insects and can be classified as phoretic or necromenic. Parasitism is another type of relationship between invertebrates and nematodes. In this case, nematodes can cause various harmful effects on insect hosts, including sterility, reduced reproductive capacity, shortened lifespan, decreased flight activity, delayed development, or other behavioral, physiological, and morphological changes.

Today, it is known that some nematodes are commercially produced to present biological control against agricultural pests. In addition to diversifying the soil fauna, diversifying with different plants that repel harmful nematodes will also be effective. Furthermore, various bacterial and fungal species that are natural antagonists against them can also be utilized.

This book will take you on a journey into the complex and mysterious world of nematodes. This journey will begin with a general overview of nematode evolution, biodiversity, and ecological roles from the past to the present, followed by a discussion of nematodes that are presented for the fight against various arthropods that damage plants for sustainable agriculture. Alongside fungi and plant species to present in effective biological control of agricultural pest nematodes, information will be shared on increasing host resistance against nematodes.

Nihal Dogan
Professor,
Medical Faculty,
Microbiology Department,
Eskisehir Osmangazi University,
Eskisehir, Turkey

Chapter 1

Round Worms from Past to Present: Evolution, Biodiversity, and Ecological Roles

Nihal Dogan

Abstract

Nematodes are one of the most diverse groups of animals on Earth. Although about 30,000 have been scientifically described, estimates suggest that the total number of species may exceed hundreds of thousands. They play important ecological roles in the plant and animal worlds, with vastly different sizes and living standards. However, many of its members are parasites that harm human and animal health and destroy agricultural products. The filamentous or cylindrical nematodes have a wide variety of habitats thanks to their advanced morphology. Some can live in or on plant roots, preventing their growth, while others live in the intestines or blood and tissues of humans and other animals, causing serious health problems. A significant number live free in soil and water, where they break down organic matter and contribute to the balance of the ecosystem. In this article, we will explore the historical development of parasitic nematodes, their diversity and importance in ecosystems, their distribution worldwide, and nematode prevention and control strategies.

Keywords: nematodes, biodiversity, blood-tissue nematodes, intestinal nematodes, plant nematodes, paleoparasitology, epidemiology, diagnosis, control

1. Introduction

Nematoda, meaning "thread" in Greek, are separate sexual creatures whose bodies consist of a single piece, round, thread-like body structures and whose sizes can be between 1 mm and 1 m, depending on the species. They have a nervous, muscular, and reproductive system, but no circulatory and respiratory systems. Their digestive system starts with the mouth and ends with anus (**Figure 1**). Females lay eggs, and some species give birth to larvae. They complete their evolution through several larval stages. During larval stages, a new cuticle layer is synthesized. Parasitic nematodes have a dauer larval stage that allows them to infect their host. In this way, they can easily resist adverse conditions. Nematodes, of which more than 30,000 species have been described to the present day, have a very crowded biodiversity. It is estimated that there are more than 1 million species, including those from prehistoric times and those that have not yet been classified today. Their mouthparts vary according to species and can be in a simple tubular or cutting-piercing style.

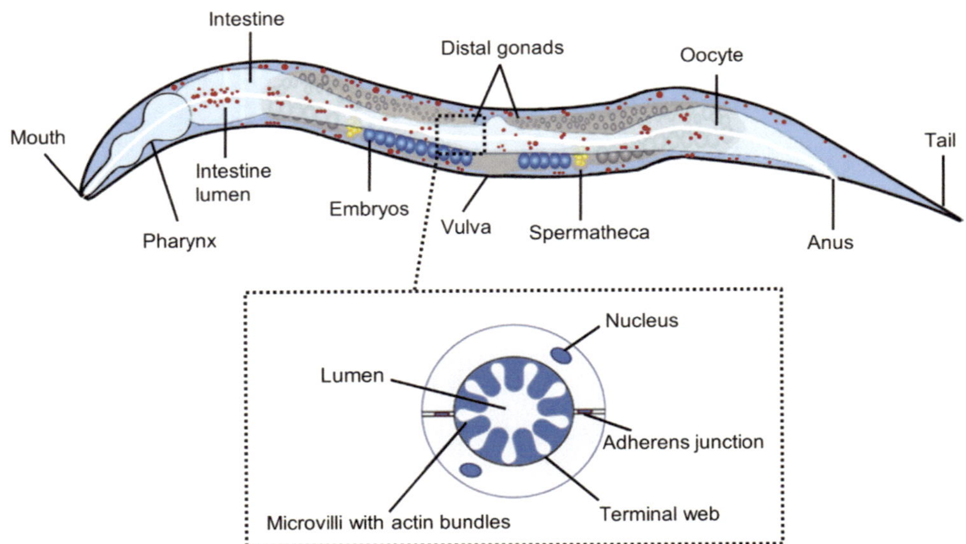

Figure 1.
General characteristics of nemathelminthes. Original source: An et al. [1].

The habitats of filamentous worms are quite diverse, ranging from humid nooks and crannies to arctic glaciers, desert dust, hot springs, and salty sea water. Parasitic nematodes are transmitted to humans and other vertebrates by the ingestion of eggs found in the external environment or by penetration of the skin by free-living larvae in the soil. Some species that live in blood and tissues are transmitted by vector arthropods. Commensalism is one of the most important associations between nematodes and insects and is often utilized in the transportation of larvae between hosts [2–6].

A substantial number of the members of the phylum Nematoda also include plant and animal parasites that cause damage to humans, animals, and cultivated crops. It is reported that half of the world's population, mainly in tropical and sub-tropical regions, is infected with gastrointestinal nematodes (GIN). A significant proportion of these are children and women [2, 3, 5, 6]. All living things in nature are easily affected by nematode attacks. For example, more than 1 million people in the world suffer physical and mental incapacitation, often ending in death, due to nematode parasitising humans. Nematodes in animals that play a role in human nutrition cause huge economic losses. Likewise, soil nematodes, which have hundreds of species, cause global damage in agriculture worldwide. Nematodes can harm plant, animal, and human health in various ways. Among these, for example, plant nematodes cause significant damage such as disrupting the structure of root cells in plants, piercing the cell wall and feeding on the cell contents, and transmitting microbial agents such as bacteria, fungi, and viruses that they carry with them to their host. More than 300 nematode species are known to affect human and animal health in tropical and sub-tropical countries, especially in developing countries. A majority of these nematodes are the so-called "soil-transmitted nematodes" and still have high morbidity and mortality rates [2–10].

In this article, we will take a brief tour through the filamentous worms. Their histories, morphological structures, species diversity, factors affecting the diversity, evolutionary processes from past to present, effects of parasitic nematodes on living organisms, life cycles and reproductive habits, interactions with other organisms, positive and negative effects on the ecosystem, developments in diagnosis-treatment and prevention measures, current developments, and current research and future perspectives will be discussed.

2. Taxonomy of nematodes

The taxonomy of nematodes, a very large group in the world, is frequently updated with innovations in diagnostic methods and the discovery of new species. In the interest of space, here we present a summary classification of the entire Phylum Nematoda based on current molecular, developmental, and morphological evidence. The classification reflects the evolutionary relationships within the branch, as well as significant areas of uncertainty, particularly with regard to the early evolution of nematodes. Only numerical diversity will be discussed here due to the large area covered. Accordingly, the Phylum Nematoda includes 2 classes, 8 subclasses, 12 superorders, 32 orders, 53 suborders, 101 superfamilies, 276 families, 511 subfamilies, 3030 genera, and 28,537 species [11–20].

How many Nematodes parasitize the Earth? The answer to this question is still not clear. Despite the developments in taxonomy, it is estimated to be about 100–350 thousand with current approaches and mathematical modeling. It is claimed that even half of the nematodes belonging to vertebrates that have been identified and collected in the world to date can be identified. Today, the power law formula is used to determine global helminth diversity. In modeling, studies have mostly focused on nematodes of vertebrates. It should be noted that there is still insufficient information on marine amphibians and reptiles. Calculations of species diversity in parasites were carried out according to certain rules. The possibility of completing this work in the twenty-first century seems difficult. For success, genome studies need to be supported by global projects [18–24].

3. History and evolution of nematodes

Nematodes are believed to have evolved from their early ancestors in the ocean, and the first animal-parasitic nematodes are thought to have parasitized marine invertebrates. Paleoparasitological studies have shown that amber, stones, and coprolites containing fossils that have reached the present day contain various evidence related to the evolution of nematodes. The oldest of these is a plant nematode from the Devonian period. Nematodes parasitizing invertebrates first appeared in the Cretaceous period, while parasitic nematodes of vertebrates have been found in Triassic coprolites. Due to the size, structure, and soft bodies of most nematodes, fossil records remain limited. Although they can be large, their rapid decomposition after death has prevented fossilization. Among the remains shedding light on the history of nematodes, amber occupies an important place. Amber, a tree resin that can protect various microorganisms and vertebrates, has allowed for a journey into the history of nematodes. However, the nematodes found in amber are primarily arthropod nematodes related to their feeding habits. A significant portion of nematodes found in humans and other vertebrates is derived from coprolites (fossilized feces) and dates back up to 240 years. In later periods, it has been possible to understand more about these organisms from fossil sources found in wetlands [5, 12, 23–32].

Nematode fossils dating back approximately 2 million years are found in Holocene deposits. Additionally, a species of *Strongyloides* associated with vertebrates has been identified in a late-stage mummified horse fossil. Research suggests that animal nematodes likely evolved in marine environments before transitioning to land. The origins of plant nematodes are believed to trace back to the Devonian period. The data provide important insights into the evolution and history of nematodes [5, 12, 23, 27, 30].

The first remains of parasitic nematodes have been identified as a plant nematode from the Early Devonian period, dating back 396 million years. Their existence marks the initial symbiotic relationships between terrestrial plants and animal organisms. The oldest animal parasitic nematodes were recently discovered in Triassic synodont coprolites in Brazil. Among these are a 240-million-year-old ascarid, *Ascarites rufferi*, and a 240-million-year-old oxyurid, *Paleoxyuris cockburni*. The next oldest member of this group is a 130-million-year-old mermithid, *Cretacimermis libani*, found in Lebanese amber from the Early Cretaceous period. A wide variety of parasitic nematodes have been found in Baltic amber. The first nematode identified in amber belongs to a species of ant and dates back to the Pliocene epoch [5, 27–32].

In Germany, freshwater accumulations in swampy areas have yielded nematode species dating back 2.5 million years, which are parasites of Tabanid flies. Various vertebrate-parasitic nematodes have been reported from deposits stretching back to the Pleistocene (up to 1.81 million years ago) and those from the Holocene era (from 11,500 BP to 3300 BC). The evolution of invertebrate nematode parasites likely first occurred with "aphasmid" nematodes in marine invertebrate hosts and later with Phasmid nematodes in terrestrial environments. Parasitic nematodes from the Cambrian period have been identified in nearshore areas.

The first evidence of nematode parasites in vertebrates has been found in freshwater habitats dating from the Cambrian period, located in nearshore regions. These findings suggest that the nematodes resided in primitive jawed organisms living in marine environments. It is proposed that modern oxyurid nematodes may represent the oldest parasites of terrestrial vertebrates. Evolutionary studies indicate that plant-parasitic nematodes have evolved at least three times, while animal-parasitic nematodes have gone through six evolutionary events [5, 19, 24, 33, 34].

Nematodes possess a broad range of vertebrate and invertebrate hosts, enabling them to transition easily between hosts and develop the ability to migrate within different organs of various hosts. Additionally, they have adapted their reproductive strategies according to their hosts. To further facilitate transitions between hosts, they have evolved attractive colors and morphological shapes. These adaptations have enhanced the evolutionary success of nematodes and allowed them to achieve widespread distribution in ecosystems [29, 31–40].

It is known that more than 4,000 plants in the world are infected with various nematodes. This situation will cause enormous agricultural damage and starvation for many people. Agricultural nematodes can also undergo continuous phylogenetic changes, facilitating their settlement in their hosts and developing genetic resistance to pesticides. Plant parasitic nematodes are divided into two groups as ectoparasites or endoparasites according to their feeding mechanisms and as resident or migratory according to their duration of persistence in their hosts. Endoparasitic nematodes, when they enter a plant, impede its normal development, disrupt the cellular structure, and create specialized feeding sites for themselves. Similarly, migratory plant-parasitic nematodes also damage the host cells through their feeding. They assist in the breakdown of plant cells by releasing peptidase inhibitors. Their active movements during migration within the host cause various degenerative changes in the host's tissues. Additionally, to evade the host's defense mechanisms, they secrete enzymes that resemble the molecular structure of the host, thereby protecting themselves from the host's defense system. Plant-parasitic nematodes cause harm in different ways, such as disrupting the synthesis of cell walls and protein structures in plants through the transfer of parasitic genes [6, 8, 23, 26, 32, 35, 41].

4. Life cycle and parasite-host relationships in nematodes

Various studies on the life cycle of parasitic and free-living nematodes with phylogenetic similarities are ongoing. Although the basic mechanism of aging has not been fully analyzed, some experimental approaches are being used. For example, mutations seem to prolong the life span. Studies show that nematodes can be grouped according to their life span. Parasitic nematodes can live for up to 15 years unless they kill their host, as in the case of hookworms. The most important reason for this is that reproduction occurs continuously rather than seasonal variability as in free-living nematodes. For example, *Enterobius vermicularis*, which has a lifespan of 2–3 weeks in the human intestine, can sustain its life in its host for years thanks to its continuous egg-laying power and auto-infections. One of the most important evolved characteristics of parasitic nematodes is their high fecundity. Parasites are usually larger and have a longer life cycle than their free-living relatives [3, 12, 15, 20].

The most important factor here is their fecundity. For example, an *Ascaris* female living in the human intestine is 20–40 cm in size and lays about 200,000 eggs per day. Parasites are usually larger and have a longer life cycle than their free-living relatives. It probably survives in the intestines for a long time. In contrast, the free-living *Caenorhabditis elegans* is 1 mm long and can lay up to 300 eggs in a lifetime of about 3 weeks. However, according to some opposing views, it is difficult to prove whether the high morbidity of some nematodes, due to their aggressive lifestyle, such as *Ascaris* and hookworms, is due to the parasite's own choice or to the death of the host. In addition, factors such as ambient temperature, foraging potential, oviposition potential, adaptation, and host immunity are other important factors affecting aging and longevity. However, current studies show that the aging process of nematodes varies depending on the state of free radicals. Therefore, it is very likely that they have a longer life cycle than free-living nematodes that depend on constant climatic changes [33, 34, 36–38].

Evolutionary studies have shown that plant parasitic nematodes have evolved at least three times and animal parasitic nematodes six times. Because they have a wide range of hosts, both vertebrate and invertebrate, they have been able to easily switch between them and migrate in different organs of different hosts. They have also been able to adapt their reproductive patterns to their hosts. Nematodes are colorless and transparent animals. Cyst nematodes develop brown to black color in their cuticle due to oxidation. In order to facilitate migration between hosts, they are able to transform into attractive colors and morphological shapes [8, 33, 34].

Many parasitic nematodes use chemical clues to find a host and establish themselves. While these are often assumed to be directly related to the host, occasionally, they are reported to originate from volatile compounds secreted by the host microbiome. These studies suggest that, instead of mutual adaptations that enable the host to better defend and the parasite to better attack, for each host and parasite, the microbiome mediating the host-parasite interaction seeks to prevent or overcome manipulation. The microbiome is an influential actor in maintaining animal and plant health and well-being and can be considered an important element in understanding host-parasite interactions, disease ecology and new disease emergence, and environmental impacts on biodiversity [26].

Parasitic nematodes, in contrast to other animals, have undergone a number of molecular and genomic adaptations during their adaptation to parasitism. The identification of these adaptations can be demonstrated experimentally by various methods. These include comparing the genomes of closely related parasitic and free-living species, comparing the gene expression of parasitic and free-living life cycle stages of parasitic nematode species, and analyzing the molecules secreted by parasitic nematodes. While many genomics-based studies on adaptation to parasitism have been conducted, there is still work to be performed given the species diversity of nematodes. Common findings in genomic-based studies are that some specialized gene families coding for proteases/peptidases, protease inhibitors, SCP/TAPS proteins, acetylcholine esterases, and so on are abundantly represented, and in most cases, these genes appear to be used and often secreted, especially during intra-host parasitic phases [8, 26, 40].

A high level of reproduction may have driven the parasite's "virulence," that is, parasite-induced host harm. Reproduction requires a large number of resources for parasites, which must come from the host. Virulence may also mean that it is a necessary part of parasitism as a consequence of the high reproductive capacity required by parasites. Nematodes are hermaphroditic and reproduce sexually, giving them an important evolutionary trait. Because of their sexual reproduction, adult nematodes do not multiply in numbers within the host. They therefore remain in the host in the same numbers as when they were acquired. Some of them are excreted by eggs and then undergo a maturation process, after which they are transmitted back to their host or pass from host to host via a vector. The lifespan of these species is directly proportional to their host. During their life in the host, they are in constant contact with their immune responses and have to develop a number of traits in order to survive. In order to protect themselves from the host defense system, they have developed features such as the ability to follow some molecules of the host, to change their own cellular structure, and to create an inflammatory response in order to protect themselves from the host defense system. These features are highly developed in nematodes living in the intestinal tract as well as in filarial nematodes living in blood and tissues. In some cases, they are also known to slow down their reproduction in order to be less affected by the host defense system. Likewise, nematodes living in the blood and lymphatic system have been shown to be sustained by secretions that attract various vertebrates as they migrate from one host to another. Parasitic nematodes have evolved in this way to maintain their species [37–40].

5. Feeding habits of parasitic nematodes

Plant and animal nematodes have a wide variety of feeding habits. Accordingly, their damages cause significant losses both in human health and in agriculture and animal husbandry. The nutritional requirements and metabolic dependence of nematodes are directly proportional to the damage they cause. In nature, there are many vertebrate and invertebrate hosts as well as a wide variety of plants that can form the feeding group of nematodes. Phylogenetic studies have suggested that plant and animal parasitic nematodes have undergone multiple evolutionary processes, resulting in a diversity of feeding habits. They have a complex life cycle and biodiversity. The complexity of their diet has led to a number of changes in the evolutionary processes of both nematodes and their hosts. All parasitic nematodes are absolutely dependent on their hosts for nutrition and energy. Considering their diversity, all living organisms in the world have been attacked by nematodes at least once in their lifetime. Nematode attacks on human essential nutrients cause global losses of millions of dollars annually. In addition, the food supply of low-income countries becomes almost impossible. Parasitic nematodes carry out this process with the support of the mouthparts they have developed as well as the various enzymes they secrete. Depending on the variety of nematodes, their food requirements may also be different. Animal parasites feed on tissue fluid and blood, while plant parasites feed on sap secretions. Studies on the different nutritional needs of nematodes are continuing [2, 3, 8, 26, 34, 36, 39, 42, 43].

The life cycles of nematodes infecting humans are quite different. Some are transmitted to the host by their larvae penetrating the skin, some are transmitted through food and water, and some are transmitted through vectors. The feeding preferences of nematodes differ according to species. Those living in the blood and tissues feed on blood, tissue, and body fluids, while those living in the intestinal system feed on intestinal contents. Since a significant number of gastrointestinal nematodes are hematophage nematodes, such as hookworms, they cause blood loss and iron deficiency in their hosts. Likewise, nematodes living in tissues feed on the muscle tissue of the host, as well as leave their larvae in muscle ligaments through the circulation. Tissue nematodes survive in the muscles of many carnivorous hosts other than humans and cause a wide diversity of symptoms. Among the tissue nematodes, Filarial nematodes are another group of vector-borne nematodes that cause permanent damage to humans and are highly prevalent in certain endemic areas around the world. While some of them cause obstruction in the lymph flow and cause overgrowth in the organs (such as *Wuchereria bancrofti, Brugia malayi, Brugia timori*), others are also vector-borne and cause river blindness disease (such as *Onchocerca volvulus, Loa loa*). More than 200 million people in endemic areas are affected by lymphatic filariasis [2, 3, 42, 43].

Plant parasitic nematodes, which are divided into two as ectoparasites or endoparasites according to their feeding mechanisms, are also divided into two as resident or migratory according to the duration of their stay in their hosts. After entering the plant, endoparasitic nematodes obstruct the normal development of the plant, destroy the cell structure, and create their own special feeding pools. Likewise, migratory plant-parasitic nematodes damage the host cell by feeding. They help plant cells to break down with the peptidase inhibitors they secrete. They cause degeneration with their active movements during migration. To protect themselves from host defense mechanisms, they secrete enzymes that resemble the molecular structure of the host. Plant parasitic nematodes damage plants in different ways, such as disrupting cell wall synthesis and protein structures by transferring parasitic genes [2, 8, 44–46].

6. Distribution of nematodes worldwide

Nematodes are the most widespread group of organisms in the world. They can therefore infect all kinds of multicellular animals and plants in all terrestrial and aquatic environments. Some authors consider parasitism by nematodes as a normal feature of life. Their biology and life cycle is an important factor in their distribution around the world. Soil-borne nematodes such as *Ascaris lumbricoides*, hookworms, *Trichuris trichiura*, and *Strongyloides stercoralis*, which are human parasites, are still among the most common parasitic infections in the tropics and subtropics worldwide [46–49].

According to WHO reports, the morbidity and mortality of these nematodes, which affect millions of people, is quite high, especially in children. Although they have decreased with sanitation and hygiene practices in developed countries, they continue to be prevalent in developing countries and rural areas due to economic and social factors. Today, these infections are still on the WHO's list of "Neglected Tropical Diseases" and are among the global health priorities. WHO has to frequently update its risk maps on the geographical distribution of nematodes according to geographical reports. Recent studies indicate a high prevalence of infection, especially in low- and middle-income countries. The situation is similar for nematodes living in blood and tissues. Despite all efforts, the prevalence of lymphatic filariasis remains high in the tropics and subtropics [46–58]. According to the latest WHO reports, 794 people in 44 countries have been treated against STHs in the last 10 years. This has led to significant reductions in the prevalence of the disease compared to previous years, but prevention and control strategies have suffered significant setbacks during the COVID-19 pandemic [54].

It is estimated that 1.5 billion people worldwide are infected with soil-transmitted helminths (STHs). Soil-transmitted helminths (STHs) are a group of intestinal parasites that are transmitted to humans through the ingestion of infective eggs or transcutaneous penetration of larvae excreted in human feces, contaminating soil and water resources. It mostly affects children in the world, especially in developing countries. It is an important source of morbidity and mortality. Distribution of nematode infections in the world's most populous countries (**Table 1**) is indicated [54].

According to the WHO 2020 reports, STHs affect 820 million people in 102 countries worldwide. Among these, the most common species are *Ascaris lumbricoides* (820 million), *Trichuris trichiura* (460 million), and hookworm infections (*Necator americanus* and *Ancylostoma duodenale*) affecting 460 million people. In addition, in 2020, serological studies in some regions reported that 386 million people had Strongyloidiasis. This nematode, which can be diagnosed by serological tests rather than fecal examinations, is estimated to be more numerous than reported. The same can be said for Toxocariasis infections. Since the diagnosis of this zoonotic nematode can only be made by serologic methods, the number is estimated to be much higher than known. In a 2019 systematic meta-analysis study, the global prevalence of Toxocariasis was defined as 19%. These rates are estimated to be higher in Africa and Southeast Asia, where serologic testing is not available [54].

In endemic areas, these rates contribute to an estimated 3.4 million disability-adjusted life years (DALYs) and 6,000 deaths. It causes developmental delay and developmental and cognitive impairment, particularly in children, due to malnutrition, fat malabsorption, vitamin malabsorption, and iron deficiency anemia. In endemic areas, multiple nematode infections can often be observed. STHs not only cause intestinal obstruction and physical and mental retardation, but they can also migrate to different organs due to migration of their larvae in the case of corticosteroid or immunosuppression for any reason, carry various microbial agents with them, and cause hyperinfection syndrome such as bacteremia and meningitis. Among these, eosinophilia and hepatitis are the most common syndromes [46, 49, 54, 58–64].

Although health education, provision of clean water, and antiparasitic treatment programs have been successful in preventing morbidity in STD control strategy programs implemented by WHO in endemic areas, they have not been fully successful

DOI: http://dx.doi.org/10.5772/intechopen.1012395

Country	Population [19]	STH[a] [20] 2012	LF [21] 2013	Schisto[a] [22] 2013	Total worms[b]	Worm index[c]	Worm index rank	HDI [6, 18]	HDI rank [6, 18]
China	1.393 billion	18.4 million	0	0.1 million	18.5 million	0.013	14	0.719	91
India	1.267 billion	170.7 million	489.1 million	0	659.8 million	0.521	6	0.586	135
USA	323 million	0	0	0	0	0	16	0.914	1
Indonesia	253 million	43.6 million	99.7 million	<0.1 million	143.3 million	0.566	5	0.684	108
Brazil	202 million	8.9 million	0.3 million	1.5 million	10.7 million	0.052	13	0.744	79
Pakistan	185 million	21.8 million	0	0	21.8 million	0.117	9	0.537	146
Nigeria	179 million	43.6 million	114.3 million	23.2 million	181.1 million	1.012	2	0.504	152
Bangladesh	159 million	31.4 million	49.7 million	0	81.1 million	0.510	7	0.558	142
Russia	142 million	0	0	0	0	0	16	0.778	57
Japan	127 million	0	0	0	0	0	16	0.890	15
Mexico	124 million	7.0 million	0	0	7.0 million	0.056	11	0.756	71
Philippines	100 million	22.2 million	19.5 million	0.5 million	42.2 million	0.422	8	0.660	117
Ethiopia	97 million	22.8 million	30 million	12.0 million	64.8 million	0.668	4	0.435	173
Vietnam	93 million	5.2 million	0	0	5.2 million	0.056	12	0.638	121
Egypt	84 million	0	0.6 million	0.1 million	0.7 million	0.008	15	0.682	110
Germany	83 million	0	0	0	0	0	16	0.911	2
Iran	78 million	0	0	0	0	0	16	0.749	75
Turkey	76 million	0	0	0	0	0	16	0.759	69
DR Congo	69 million	19.6 million	49.1 million	10.2 million	78.9 million	1.143	1	0.338	186

Country	Population [19]	STH[a] [20] 2012	LF [21] 2013	Schisto[a] [22] 2013	Total worms[b]	Worm index[c]	Worm index rank	HDI [6, 18]	HDI rank [6, 18]
Thailand	67 million	0	0	0	0	0	16	0.722	89
France	65 million	0	0	0	0	0	16	0.884	20
United Kingdom	63 million	0	0	0	0	0	16	0.892	3
Italy	61 million	0	0	0	0	0	16	0.872	26
Burma	54 million	8.1 million	39.5 million	0	47.6 million	0.881	3	0.524	150
South Africa	53 million	2.3 million	0	2.5 million	4.8 million	0.090	10	0.658	118
Total	5.4 billion				1.37 billion	0.254		0.702	

[a] *Data for school-aged children only.*
[b] *Calculated by adding columns 3–5.*
[c] *Calculated by dividing number of total worm infections obtained in column 6 by population in column 2.*
doi:10.1371/journal.pntd.0003618.t001.

Table 1.
Distribution of nematode infections in the world's most populous countries. Source: https://www.who.int/publications/i/item/9789240000315.

due to other outbreaks, economic inadequacies, and labor deficits from time to time. Increased global migration to developed countries due to climate change has led to the emergence of Neglected Tropical Diseases (NTDs) in non-endemic countries. With increased global migration, people infected with NTDs may move to countries where these diseases are not present. This can lead to difficulties and delays in diagnosis and treatment of infection [58–64].

7. Diagnostic methods in nematodes

The diagnosis of nematodes in the intestinal tract is made by macroscopic and microscopic examination of feces. Since these nematodes, most of which are of soil origin, have a larval migration period shortly after infection, larvae can be searched for in sputum and vomit samples during this period. To increase the chance of finding nematode eggs, feces should be prepared by sedimentation. Here, methods such as Kato-Katz, Wisconsin flotation, and Haroda-Mori increase the chance of detection. These methods have their own positive and negative advantages and disadvantages [65, 66].

Molecular methods allow for better species identification of many nematodes. However, their use is limited by the need for a variety of equipment. Serologic tests for nematode coproantigens are not suitable for field work due to low sensitivity and specificity and cannot distinguish whether infection is present or past. ELISA and Latex tests are among the tests used in field studies, but their specificity is low due to the common antigenic structure of nematodes. In large-scale epidemiological studies, samples are mostly collected and used for PCR applications in specific laboratories [67, 68].

In the diagnosis of soil-transmitted nematodes, high eosinophilia in blood parameters and mild or severe anemia are also common signs of infections. Helminths should be considered in the presence of Charcot-Leyden crystals in stool and sputum and the presence of fecal occult blood. Colonoscopy is important in the diagnosis as whipworms are located in the rectum [69, 70].

Similar practices are also practiced in veterinary parasitology. In addition to microscopic examination, immunodiagnostic methods are also used for rapid diagnosis. Recently, in addition to rapid and reliable methods, quantifiable molecular and immunodiagnostic methods such as artificial intelligence have been used to perform the necessary examination in a large number of farm animals. However, due to the variability of reproductive cycles of nematodes with different evolutionary cycles, the results are not always successful. In addition, microscopic diagnosis requires experience [71, 72].

Investigating the presence of plant nematodes is very difficult as large areas need to be investigated. Statistical methods are mostly used to describe their quantity or presence. The results obtained by examining samples of soil or plant samples scanned by random sampling methods in large areas of cultivated land are calculated by statistical methods. Research on agricultural nematodes is important in terms of determining damage and identifying species diversity, population trends, soil types, and climate changes. For this purpose, 250–300 ml of soil samples around the cultivated roots in agricultural fields are placed in polyethylene bags, and the necessary data are noted. The collected samples should be extracted and analyzed in a short time. Extraction processes are applied according to various techniques. After the samples are prepared according to the enrichment method, they are examined by microscopy, serological, or molecular methods using various methods. Biological, biochemical, and cytogenetic methods are used to identify some plant nematodes. In this way, their taxonomy is also made [72–74].

8. Treatment, prevention, and control strategies for nematodes

Unfortunately, the number of drugs used in the treatment of nematodes has been limited to a small number of drugs from the past to the present. Today, the development of resistance to anthelmintics is quite common. Due to the development of economic and anthelmintic resistance, there are great losses due to parasitic nematodes in various animal groups and agricultural products in different geographies of the world [75–77].

Today STHs infections are still the most prevalent of neglected tropical diseases, primarily affecting child populations in low- and middle-income countries. In these areas, more than 1 billion people are infected with STHs. WHO has announced that significant success has been achieved with chemotherapy in risk groups consisting of pre-school, school age, and women of childbearing age by 2020 with the control program launched in 2012. The organization has decided to continue prevention and control practices until 2030 to ensure the success of the work.

It proposes an integrated approach that includes access to proper sanitation, hygiene education, and preventive chemotherapy (large-scale and periodic distribution of anthelminthic drugs). To this end, WHO has been providing Benzimidazole treatment in endemic areas with donors since 2010. Approximately 4 billion Benzimidazole treatments have been given in schools, and significant reductions in morbidity have been reported. Treatment and monitoring of lymphatic filariasis is also being implemented in the same areas. Donors are needed to ensure the success of preventive treatment programs in endemic areas [75–79].

In recent years, some countries have been searching for alternative prevention methods against the development of resistance and side effects of drugs. Biological methods used as alternative methods will prevent human-animal and environmental damage. Nematophages, the natural competitors of nematodes, are potential biological control agents like microbes. These natural enemies include both bacteria and fungi and use a variety of methods to infect and kill nematodes. For example, nematode-capturing fungi can sense host signals and produce specialized capture devices to capture nematodes, while endo-parasitic fungi can kill nematodes through spore adhesion and invasive growth to break the nematode cuticle [79–82].

It should also be able to prevent transmission and prevent various complications with simple measures to be taken. Personal hygiene, clean water, sewage and treatment systems, cooking and consumption of food, public education, and improvement of living conditions are extremely important criteria for elimination. It is important that individuals in risk groups (children, pet owners) are periodically checked by a doctor [54, 77, 80].

The cost of praziquantel and other anthelmintics has decreased to such an extent that the cost should no longer prevent epidemic countries from easily delivering them to those in need. Regular treatment can be provided in an affordable and sustainable way with available medicines. This strategy, aimed at reaching those at the highest risk of morbidity from schistosomiasis and soil-transmitted helminthiasis, was endorsed by the World Health Assembly in May 2001 [83, 84].

From the past to the present, according to WHO criteria, people diagnosed with geo helminths must receive antihelminthic treatment. The prevalence has decreased considerably in many countries due to antihelminthic treatment since the 1970s. Nowadays, oral rehydration is an important step in the treatment in order to make the treatment more successful. Treatment reduces parasite load and complications and prevents transmission. In endemic areas, treatment is recommended to be repeated every 6 months or once a year to prevent new infections.

Prevention and control strategies for nematodes have not yet achieved the desired success. It is necessary to facilitate community access to anthelmintics and to make them available to the widest masses. In addition, there is a need for the discovery of new drugs with fewer side effects and that are more economical. However, treating soil-borne nematodes with drugs alone may not be a permanent solution because vaccination seems to be a better way for elimination due to the high rates of re-infection [78–88].

9. Challenges, solution, and future expectations

Nematoda is a large group of plant and animal parasites that cause significant damage to humans and agricultural crops. The most extensive studies of members of this group have focused on human, animal, and agricultural pests. It is estimated that about half of the world's human population is infected with nematodes. Parasitic nematodes have to constantly modify their individual life cycles in order to live long lives with their hosts. Their life history suggests that the process of future evolution is still ongoing. The appearance of nematode infections in different geographical regions is an important indicator of this. Factors such as various climatic changes and migration of human populations from one place to another for various reasons and tourism also contribute to this diversity and evolution. In addition, one of the most important evolutions is the resistance they have developed against various antiparasitic drugs used for therapeutic purposes. In the twenty-first century, nematodes are still an important source of morbidity and mortality in children in certain areas of the world. According to WHO's target, solutions, such as finding donors and establishing training guidelines and rapid and effective diagnosis and treatment methods have been planned to control SHTs by 2030. However, increasing economic problems make it difficult to find donors, and control is becoming increasingly difficult due to other epidemics, wars, and migrations.

A type of roundworms, nematodes are widespread throughout the world, and a significant number of them are free-living in nature. Some live in freshwater, some in the oceans, and some in the soil. They decompose various harmful microorganisms that they use to feed on and transform them into useful ones. They decompose organic matter and transform it into something useful for soil and agricultural plants. They contribute to biological control by consuming many harmful parasites. They are an important model in genetic research. Nematodes are indispensable elements of nature's complex and balanced ecosystems. Their evolutionary processes, diversity, and ecological roles have had a profound impact on both natural and human life. Understanding them is of great importance both in terms of biodiversity and in the fields of sustainable agriculture and health. Getting rid of their harmful effects requires the collective fight against them.

Author details

Nihal Dogan
Faculty of Medical, Department of Microbiology, Eskişehir Osmangazi University, Turkey

*Address all correspondence to: nihaldogan42@gmail.com and ndogan@ogu.edu.tr

References

[1] An L, Fu X, Chen J, Ma J. Application of *Caenorhabditis elegans* in lipid metabolism research. Int J Mol Sci. 2023;**24**(2):1173. DOI: 10.3390/ijms24021173

[2] Lin CJ, Siddique S. Parasitic nematodes: Dietary habits and their implications. Trends in Parasitology. 2024;**40**(3):230-240. DOI: 10.1016/j.pt.2023.12.013. Epub 2024 Jan 22

[3] Kiontke K, Fitch DH. Nematodes. Current Biology. 2013;**23**(19):R862-R864. DOI: 10.1016/j.cub.2013.08.009

[4] Vlaar LE, Bertran A, Rahimi M, Dong L, Kammenga JE, Helder J, et al. On the role of dauer in the adaptation of nematodes to a parasitic lifestyle. Parasites & Vectors. 2021;**14**(1):554. DOI: 10.1186/s13071-021-04953-6

[5] Poinar GO Jr. The geological record of parasitic nematode evolution. Advances in Parasitology. 2015;**90**:53-92. DOI: 10.1016/bs.apar.2015.03.002. Epub 2015 Apr 15

[6] Powers TO, Harris TS, Higgins RS, Mullin PG, Powers KS. Nematode biodiversity assessments need vouchered databases: A BOLD reference library for plant-parasitic nematodes in the superfamily Criconematoidea. Genome. 2021;**64**(3):232-241. DOI: 10.1139/gen-2019-0196. Epub 2020 Jun 11

[7] Bird DM, Jones JT, Opperman CH, Kikuchi T, Danchin EG. Signatures of adaptation to plant parasitism in nematode genomes. Parasitology. 2015;**142**(Suppl. 1):S71-S84. DOI: 10.1017/S0031182013002163

[8] Dayi M. Diversity and evolution of transposable elements in the plant-parasitic nematodes. BMC Genomics. 2024;**25**(1):511. DOI: 10.1186/s12864-024-10435-7

[9] Khazaei M, Parsasefat M, Bahar A, Tahmasebi H, Oksenych V. Behavioral cooperation or conflict of human intestinal roundworms and microbiomes: A bio-activity perspective. Cells. 2025;**14**(7):556. DOI: 10.3390/cells14070556

[10] Ryss AY. Evolution of life cycles of nematodes parasitizing woody plants As a result of ecological and phylogenetic co-adaptations with hosts and vectors. Doklady. Biochemistry and Biophysics. 2024;**518**(1):325-345. DOI: 10.1134/S1607672924701047. Epub 2024 Jul 1

[11] Machado RAR, Von Reuss SH. Chemical ecology of nematodes. Chimia (Aarau). 2022;**76**(11):945-953. DOI: 10.2533/chimia.2022.945

[12] Ferreıra LF, Reınhard KJ, Araújo A, editors. Foundations of Paleoparasitology [Online]. Rio de Janeiro: Editora FIOCRUZ; 2014. 462 p. DOI: 10.7476/9788575415986. ISBN: 978-85-7541-598-6. Available from: http://books.scielo.org/id/zngnn/epub/ferreira-9788575415986.epub

[13] Moser MS, Hallem EA. Astacin metalloproteases in human-parasitic nematodes. Advances in Parasitology. 2024;**126**:177-204. DOI: 10.1016/bs.apar.2024.03.001. Epub 2024 Apr 14

[14] Veesenmeyer AF. Important nematodes in children. Pediatric Clinics of North America. 2022;**69**(1):129-139. DOI: 10.1016/j.pcl.2021.08.005

[15] Cole R, Viney M. The population genetics of parasitic nematodes of wild animals. Parasit Vectors. 2018;**11**(1):590.

DOI: 10.1186/s13071-018-3137-5. Erratum in: Parasites & Vectors 2019 Oct 9; 12(1):468. doi: 10.1186/s13071-019-3731-1

[16] Hodda M. Phylum Nematoda: A classification, catalogue and index of valid genera, with a census of valid species. Zootaxa. 2022;**5114**(1):1-289. DOI: 10.11646/zootaxa.5114.1.1

[17] Denver DR, Clark KA, Raboin MJ. Reproductive mode evolution in nematodes: Insights from molecular phylogenies and recently discovered species. Molecular Phylogenetics and Evolution. 2011;**61**(2):584-592. DOI: 10.1016/j.ympev.2011.07.007. Epub 2011 Jul 20

[18] Blaxter ML. Nematoda: Genes, genomes and the evolution of parasitism. Advances in Parasitology. 2003;**54**:101-195. DOI: 10.1016/s0065-308x(03)54003-9

[19] Jackson AP. Preface. The evolution of parasite genomes and the origins of parasitism. Parasitology. 2015;**142**(Suppl. 1):S1-S5. DOI: 10.1017/S0031182014001516

[20] Carlson CJ, Dallas TA, Alexander LW, Phelan AL, Phillips AJ. What would it take to describe the global diversity of parasites? Proceedings of the Biological Sciences. 1939;**2020**(287):20201841. DOI: 10.1098/rspb.2020.1841. Epub 2020 Nov 18

[21] Strona G, Fattorini S. Parasitic worms: How many really? International Journal for Parasitology. 2014;**44**(5):269-272. DOI: 10.1016/j.ijpara.2014.01.002. Epub 2014 Feb 14

[22] Shapiro JT, Víquez-R L, Leopardi S, Vicente-Santos A, Mendenhall IH, Frick WF, et al. Setting the terms for zoonotic diseases: Effective communication for research, conservation, and public policy. Viruses. 2021;**13**(7):1356. DOI: 10.3390/v13071356

[23] Blaxter M, Koutsovoulos G. The evolution of parasitism in Nematoda. Parasitology. 2015;**142**(Suppl. 1):S26-S39. DOI: 10.1017/S0031182014000791. Epub 2014 Jun 25

[24] Leung TL. Fossils of parasites: What can the fossil record tell us about the evolution of parasitism? Biological Reviews of the Cambridge Philosophical Society. 2017;**92**(1):410-430. DOI: 10.1111/brv.12238. Epub 2015 Nov 5

[25] Kornobis FW. Typy troficzne nicieni [Trophic types of the nematodes]. Wiadomości Parazytologiczne. 2008;**54**(1):1-9. Polish

[26] Speer KA. Microbiomes mediate host-parasite interactions. Molecular Ecology. 2022;**31**(7):1925-1927. DOI: 10.1111/mec.16381. Epub 2022 Feb 19

[27] Borba VH, Machado-Silva JR, Le Bailly M, Iniguez AM. Worldwide paleodistribution of capillariid parasites: Paleoparasitology, current status of phylogeny and taxonomic perspectives. PLoS ONE. 2019;**14**(4):e0216150

[28] De Baets K, Vanadzina K, Schiffbauer J. Trapped in time. eLife. 2023;**12**:e90008. DOI: 10.7554/eLife.90008

[29] Campião KM, Morais DH, Dias OT, Aguiar A, Toledo Gde M, Tavares LE, et al. Checklist of helminth parasites of amphibians from South America. Zootaxa. 2014;**3843**:1-93. DOI: 10.11646/zootaxa.3843.1.1

[30] Hugot JP, Gardner SL, Borba V, Araujo P, Leles D, Stock Da-Rosa ÁA, et al. Discovery of a 240 million year old nematode parasite egg in a cynodont coprolite sheds light on the early origin

of pinworms in vertebrates. Parasites & Vectors. 2014;**7**:486. DOI: 10.1186/s13071-014-0486-6

[31] Poinar GO Jr. The range of life in amber: Significance and implications in DNA studies. Experientia. 1994;**50**(6): 536-542. DOI: 10.1007/BF01921722

[32] van den Hoogen J, Geisen S, Wall DH, Wardle DA, Traunspurger W, de Goede RGM, et al. A global database of soil nematode abundance and functional group composition. Scientific Data. 2020;**7**(1):103. DOI: 10.1038/s41597-020-0437-3

[33] Morand S, Krasnov BR, Littlewood DTJ, editors. Parasite Diversity and Diversification: Evolutionary Ecology Meets Phylogenetics. Cambridge Univ Press; The University of Chicago Press Books: 2015. DOI: 10.1086/690864

[34] Gems D. Longevity and ageing in parasitic and free-living nematodes. Biogerontology. 2000;**1**(4):289-307. DOI: 10.1023/a:1026546719091

[35] Eves-van den Akker S. Plant-nematode interactions. Current Opinion in Plant Biology. 2021;**62**:102035. DOI: 10.1016/j.pbi.2021.102035. Epub 2021 Mar 27

[36] Nisbet AJ, Cottee PA, Gasser RB. Genomics of reproduction in nematodes: Prospects for parasite intervention? Trends in Parasitology. 2008;**24**(2):89-95. DOI: 10.1016/j.pt.2007.12.001. Epub 2008 Jan 7

[37] Rudolf VH, Lafferty KD. Stage structure alters how complexity affects stability of ecological networks. Ecology Letters. 2011;**14**(1):75-79. DOI: 10.1111/j.1461-0248.2010.01558.x. Epub 2010 Nov 30

[38] Benesh DP, Parker G, Chubb JC. Life-cycle complexity in helminths: What are the benefits? Evolution. 2021;**75**(8):1936-1952. DOI: 10.1111/evo.14299. Epub 2021 Jul 13

[39] Benesh DP, Chubb JC, Parker GA. Adaptive division of growth and development between hosts in helminths with two-host life cycles. Evolution. 2022;**76**(9):1971-1985. DOI: 10.1111/evo.14574. Epub 2022 Jul 27

[40] Viney M. The genomic basis of nematode parasitism. Briefings in Functional Genomics. 2018;**17**(1):8 14. DOI: 10.1093/bfgp/elx010

[41] Nihal D. Intestinal Parasites from Past to Present: Taxonomy, Paleoparasitology, Geographic Distribution, Prevention and Control Strategies. London, United Kingdom: W1W 5PF; 2024. ISBN: 978-0-85466-571-6. DOI: 10.5772/intechopen.1002145

[42] Lourens GB, Ferrell DK. Lymphatic Filariasis. The Nursing Clinics of North America. 2019;**54**(2):181-192. DOI: 10.1016/j.cnur.2019.02.007. Epub 2019 Mar 27

[43] Hotterbeekx A, Perneel J, Vieri MK, Colebunders R, Kumar-Singh S. The secretome of filarial nematodes and its role in host-parasite interactions and pathogenicity in onchocerciasis-associated epilepsy. Frontiers in Cellular and Infection Microbiology. 2021;**11**:662766. DOI: 10.3389/fcimb.2021.662766

[44] Viney M, Cable J. Macroparasite life histories. Current Biology. 2011;**21**(18):R767-R774. DOI: 10.1016/j.cub.2011.07.023

[45] Zarowiecki M, Berriman M. What helminth genomes have taught us about parasite evolution. Parasitology. 2015;**142**(Suppl. 1):S85-S97. DOI: 10.1017/S0031182014001449. Epub 2014 Dec 8

[46] Buonfrate D, Bisanzio D, Giorli G, Odermatt P, Fürst T, Greenaway C, et al. The global prevalence of *Strongyloides stercoralis* infection. Pathogens. 2020;**9**(6):468. DOI: 10.3390/pathogens9060468

[47] Montresor A, King JD. Elimination of lymphatic filariasis in Loa loa areas. The Lancet Infectious Diseases. 2017;**17**(7):683-684. DOI: 10.1016/S1473-3099(17)30163-9. Epub 2017 Mar 31

[48] Hotez PJ, Herricks JR. Helminth elimination in the pursuit of sustainable development goals: A "worm index" for human development. PLoS Neglected Tropical Diseases. 2015;**9**(4):e0003618. DOI: 10.1371/journal. pntd.0003618

[49] Gildner TE, Cepon-Robins TJ, Urlacher SS. Cumulative host energetic costs of soil-transmitted helminth infection. Trends in Parasitology. 2022;**38**(8):629-641. DOI: 10.1016/j.pt.2022.04.007. Epub 2022 May 19

[50] Ng'etich AI, Amoah ID, Bux F, Kumari S. Anthelmintic resistance in soil-transmitted helminths: One-health considerations. Parasitology Research. 2023;**123**(1):62. DOI: 10.1007/s00436-023-08088-8

[51] Montresor A, Garba A. Treatment of preschool children for schistosomiasis. The Lancet Global Health. 2017;**5**(7):e640-e641. DOI: 10.1016/S2214-109X(17)30202-4

[52] José MV, Ruiz A, Bobadilla JR. Prevalence of infection, mean worm burden and degree of worm aggregation as determinants of prevalence of disease due to intestinal helminths. Archives of Medical Research. 1997;**28**(1):121-127

[53] Naish S, McCarthy J, Williams GM. Prevalence, intensity and risk factors for soil-transmitted helminth infection in a south Indian fishing village. Acta Tropica. 2004;**91**(2):177-187. DOI: 10.1016/j.actatropica.2004.04.004

[54] WHO Team. p. 8. Reference Number: WHA63.16. CC BY-NC-SA 3.0 IGO. Available from: https://www.who.int/publications/i/item/who-global-code-of-practice-on-the-international-recruitment-of-health-personnel

[55] Fleitas PE, Travacio M, Martí-Soler H, Socías ME, Lopez WR, Krolewiecki AJ. The Strongyloides stercoralis-hookworms association as a path to the estimation of the global burden of strongyloidiasis: A systematic review. PLoS Neglected Tropical Diseases. 2020;**14**(4):e0008184. DOI: 10.1371/journal.pntd.0008184

[56] Yang R, Xu M, Zhang L, Liao Y, Liu Y, Deng X, et al. Human *Strongyloides stercoralis* infection. Journal of Microbiology, Immunology, and Infection. 2025;**58**(2):164-179. DOI: 10.1016/j.jmii.2024.07.010. Epub 2024 Aug 3

[57] Owjinezhad D, Abdoli A, Rahmanian V, Shaterian N, Bahadory S, Matin S, et al. Global seroprevalence of Toxocara spp. in children: A systematic review and meta-analysis. Acta Parasitologica. 2024;**69**(1):164-174. DOI: 10.1007/s11686-023-00772-0. Epub 2024 Jan 9

[58] Ahiadorme M, Morhe E. Soil transmitted helminth infections in Ghana: A ten year review. The Pan African Medical Journal. 2020;**35**:131. DOI: 10.11604/pamj.2020.35.131.21069

[59] Garn JV, Wilkers JL, Meehan AA, Pfadenhauer LM, Burns J, Imtiaz R, et al. Interventions to improve water, sanitation, and hygiene for preventing soil-transmitted helminth infection. Cochrane Database of Systematic

Reviews. 2022;**6**(6):CD012199. DOI: 10.1002/14651858.CD012199.pub2

[60] WHO Control of Neglected Tropical Diseases. 2024. Available from: https://www.who.int/teams/control-of-neglected-tropical-diseases/advocacy/

[61] Montresor A, Mwinzi P, Mupfasoni D, Garba A. Reduction in DALYs lost due to soil-transmitted helminthiases and schistosomiasis from 2000 to 2019 is parallel to the increase in coverage of the global control programmes. PLoS Neglected Tropical Diseases. 2022;**16**(7):e0010575

[62] World Health Organization. World Health Organization Factsheet on Soil-Transmitted Helminths. 2023. 2024. Available from: https://www.who.int/news-room/fact-sheets/detail/soil-transmitted-helminth-infections

[63] Purkiss J, Pepe P, Poplawski NAK, Maurelli MP, Gualdieri L, Rinaldi L, et al. Combining country indicators and individual variables to predict soil-transmitted helminth infections among migrant populations: A case study from southern Italy. PLoS Neglected Tropical Diseases. 2025;**19**(6):e0012577. DOI: 10.1371/journal.pntd.0012577

[64] Imalele EE, Braide EI, Emanghe UE, Effanga EO, Usang AU. Soil-transmitted helminth infection among school-age children in Ogoja, Nigeria: Implication for control. Parasitology Research. 2023;**122**(4):1015-1026. DOI: 10.1007/s00436-023-07809-3. Epub 2023 Mar 8

[65] Bosch F, Palmeirim MS, Ali SM, Ame SM, Hattendorf J, Keiser J. Diagnosis of soil-transmitted helminths using the Kato-Katz technique: What is the influence of stirring, storage time and storage temperature on stool sample egg counts? PLoS Neglected Tropical Diseases. 2021;**15**(1):e0009032. DOI: 10.1371/journal.pntd.0009032

[66] Dryden MW, Payne PA, Ridley R, Smith V. Comparison of common fecal flotation techniques for the recovery of parasite eggs and oocysts. Veterinary Therapeutics. 2005;**6**:15-28

[67] L'Ollivier C, Piarroux R. Diagnosis of human nematode infections. Expert Review of Anti-Infective Therapy. 2013;**11**(12):1363-1376. DOI: 10.1586/14787210.2013.851001. Epub 2013 Nov 4

[68] McKeand JB. Molecular diagnosis of parasitic nematodes. Parasitology. 1998;**117**(Suppl.):S87-S96. DOI: 10.1017/s0031182099004096

[69] Tchuem Tchuenté LA. Control of soil-transmitted helminths in sub-Saharan Africa: Diagnosis, drug efficacy concerns and challenges. Acta Tropica. 2011;**120**(Suppl. 1):S4-S11. DOI: 10.1016/j.actatropica.2010.07.001. Epub 2010 Jul 21

[70] Meulah B, Bengtson M, Lieshout LV, Hokke CH, Kreidenweiss A, Diehl JC, et al. A review on innovative optical devices for the diagnosis of human soil-transmitted helminthiasis and schistosomiasis: From research and development to commercialization. Parasitology. 2023;**150**(2):137-149. DOI: 10.1017/S0031182022001664. Epub 2022 Dec 9

[71] Rinaldi L, Krücken J, Martinez-Valladares M, Pepe P, Maurelli MP, de Queiroz C, et al. Advances in diagnosis of gastrointestinal nematodes in livestock and companion animals. Advances in Parasitology. 2022;**118**:85-176. DOI: 10.1016/bs.apar.2022.07.002. Epub 2022 Sep 2

[72] Tintori SC, Sloat SA, Rockman MV. Rapid isolation of wild nematodes by Baermann funnel. Journal of Visualized

Experiments. 31 Jan 2022;(179):63287. DOI: 10.3791/63287

[73] Maqbool MA. Plant Nematode Problems and their Control in the Near East Region (FAO Plant Production and Protection Paper - 144). Rome: Food[Z1] and Agriculture Organization of the United Nations; 1997. ISBN: 92-5-103798-1. Available from: https://www.fao.org/4/v9978e/v9978e00.htm

[74] Kikuchi T, Eves-van den Akker S, Jones JT. Genome evolution of plant-parasitic nematodes. Annual Review of Phytopathology. 2017;**55**:333-354. DOI: 10.1146/annurev-phyto-080516-035434. Epub 2017 Jun 7

[75] Montresor A, Mupfasoni D, Mikhailov A, Mwinzi P, Lucianez A, Jamsheed M, et al. The global progress of soil-transmitted helminthiases control in 2020 and World Health Organization targets for 2030. PLoS Neglected Tropical Diseases. 2020;**14**(8):e0008505

[76] Seesao Y, Gay M, Merlin S, Viscogliosi E, Aliouat-Denis CM, Audebert C. A review of methods for nematode identification. Journal of Microbiological Methods. 2017;**138**:37-49. DOI: 10.1016/j.mimet.2016.05.030. Epub 2016 Jun 2

[77] Control of Neglected Tropical Diseases (NTD). World Health Organization. p. 86. ISBN: 978-92-4-009153-5. Available from: https://www.who.int/publications/i/item/9789240091535

[78] Keenan JD, Hotez PJ, Amza A, Stoller NE, Gaynor BD, Porco TC, et al. Elimination and eradication of neglected tropical diseases with mass drug administrations: A survey of experts. PLoS Neglected Tropical Diseases. 2013;**7**(12):e2562. DOI: 10.1371/journal.pntd.0002562

[79] Muchiut SM, Fernández AS, Steffan PE, Riva E, Fiel CA. Anthelmintic resistance: Management of parasite refugia for Haemonchus contortus through the replacement of resistant with susceptible populations. Veterinary Parasitology. 2018;**254**:43-48. DOI: 10.1016/j.vetpar.2018.03.004. Epub 2018 Mar 5

[80] WHO (World Health Organization). Prevention and Control of Schistomiasis and Soil-Transmitted Helminthiasis. WHO Team; 2002. p. 57. ISBN: 92 4 120912 7. WHO reference number TRS No912. CC BY-NC-SA 3.0 IGO. Available from: https://www.who.int/publications/i/item/WHO-TRS-912

[81] Reynoldson JA, Behnke JM, Pallant LJ, Macnish MG, Gilbert F, Giles S, et al. Failure of pyrantel in treatment of human hookworm infections (*Ancylostoma duodenale*) in the Kimberley region of north West Australia. Acta Tropica. 1997;**68**:301-312

[82] Geerts S, Gryseels B. Anthelmintic resistance in human helminths: A review. Tropical Medicine & International Health. 2001;**6**:915-921

[83] World Health Assembly, 54. Fifty-Fourth World Health Assembly, Geneva, 14-22 May 2001: Resolutions and Decisions. World Health Organization; 2001. Available from: https://iris.who.int/handle/10665/260183

[84] Savioli L, Albonico M, Engels D, Montresor A. Progress in the prevention and control of schistosomiasis and soil-transmitted helminthiasis. Parasitology International. 2004;**53**(2):103-113. DOI: 10.1016/j.parint.2004.01.001

[85] Liang LM, Zou CG, Xu J, Zhang KQ. Signal pathways involved in microbe-nematode interactions provide new insights into the biocontrol of plant-parasitic nematodes. Philosophical

Transactions of the Royal Society of London. Series B, Biological Sciences. 2019;**374**(1767):20180317. DOI: 10.1098/rstb.2018.0317

[86] Kaplan RM. Biology, epidemiology, diagnosis, and management of anthelmintic resistance in gastrointestinal nematodes of livestock. The Veterinary Clinics of North America. Food Animal Practice. 2020;**36**(1):17-30. DOI: 10.1016/j.cvfa.2019.12.001

[87] 1 st ed. CRC Press; 2002. p. 19. e Book ISBN: 9780429095382. Available from: https://www.taylorfrancis.com/chapters/edit/10.1201/b12614-24/epidemiology-control-nematode-infection-disease-humans-donald-bundy-helen-guyatt-edwin-michael

[88] Loukas A, Maizels RM, Hotez PJ. The yin and yang of human soil-transmitted helminth infections. International Journal for Parasitology. 2021;**51**(13-14):1243-1253. DOI: 10.1016/j.ijpara.2021.11.001. Epub 2021 Nov 10

Chapter 2

Entomopathogenic Nematode: A Sustainable Option for IPM

Thattankandy Meethal Aparna, Mukesh R. Siddhapara and Sonam Kumari

Abstract

The chapter provides a comprehensive overview of entomopathogenic nematodes (EPNs) as viable biocontrol agents in biointensive pest management systems, particularly in the context of sustainable agriculture. Despite the underdeveloped biopesticide market, the capabilities of entomopathogenic nematodes to combat various insect pests, including those in the orders Coleoptera, Diptera, Lepidoptera, and Hemiptera, are highlighted. The chapter discusses the historical context of entomopathogenic nematode discovery, their symbiotic relationships with bacteria, and the methodologies for their isolation and mass production, including both *in vivo* and *in vitro* methods. The efficacy of various entomopathogenic nematode species against target pests is substantiated through laboratory studies and field, demonstrating significant mortality rates across multiple pest species. Additionally, the functional compatibility of entomopathogenic nematodes with chemical pesticides and entomopathogens is examined, suggesting their integrative role in pest management strategies. The findings underscore the ecological benefits of using entomopathogenic nematodes as a sustainable alternative to synthetic pesticides, emphasizing their safety for non-target organisms and humans. Overall, the study advocates for the integration of entomopathogenic nematodes into integrated pest management practices to boost pest control efficacy and promote sustainable agricultural practices in India.

Keywords: *in vivo* and *in vitro* multiplication, EPN, mass production, symbiotic bacteria, infective juveniles, IPM, mortality, biological control

1. Introduction

Despite initial expectations, the biopesticide sector in India has experienced limited growth and continues to occupy a relatively smaller share compared to the synthetic pesticide market. This slower development is attributed to various industrial and policy-related obstacles that have constrained production capacity. However, efforts to promote biopesticides as part of sustainable agricultural practices have been reinforced by initiatives such as the National Farmer Policy of 2007 [1].

The biopesticides market was valued at approximately USD 7.3 billion in 2023 and is projected to grow from USD 8.32 billion in 2024 to USD 23.74 billion by 2032, exhibiting a compound annual growth rate (CAGR) of 14.0% during the forecast period

(2025–2032). As of November 2024, a total of 970 biopesticides have been registered with the Central Insecticides Board and Registration Committee (CIBRC) under the Government of India [2]. It is estimated that by 2050, biopesticides will constitute up to 50% of the Indian pesticide market [1], a significant increase from their current share of approximately 9% of total pesticide consumption [3]. An annual growth rate of 2.5% is anticipated for the sector. Nevertheless, at present, the biopesticide market remains underdeveloped relative to initial expectations and continues to represent a modest segment compared to the synthetic pesticide industry. Production remains comparatively limited, largely due to persistent challenges at both industrial and policy levels.

Scientific evidence shows that in modern industrial agriculture, the use of synthetic pesticides contributes significantly to greenhouse gas emissions (US Environment Protection Agency 2022 [4]) and also makes our agricultural systems more vulnerable to the effects of climate change [5, 6]. Pesticides contribute to climate change throughout their entire life cycle, through production, packaging, transportation, application, and even environmental degradation and disposal [7].

Integrated Pest Management (IPM) is an ecosystem-based approach to pest control that combines multiple practices to maintain pest populations below economic threshold levels. In recent years, the incorporation of entomopathogenic nematodes (EPNs) as a component of IPM strategies has gained increasing attention, primarily to mitigate issues such as insecticide resistance, pest resurgence, and pesticide residue accumulation. Entomopathogenic nematodes (derived from 'entomo' meaning insect, and 'pathogenic' meaning disease-causing) are microscopic, soil-dwelling roundworms capable of infecting and killing insect pests. These nematodes utilize symbiotic bacteria to cause lethal infections in their hosts, making them effective biological control agents within sustainable pest management frameworks.

EPNs are exempt from registration and regulatory requirements by the United States Environmental Protection Agency (EPA), the Central Insecticides Board and Registration Committee (CIBRC) of India, and analogous regulatory bodies in several other countries.

Various biocontrol applications have used entomopathogenic nematodes as control agent [8], with inundative biological control forming the largest [9, 10]. In inundative biological control, large numbers of nematodes are released to invade the pest population and achieve immediate pest suppression [9]. Such control measures have been successfully used in field treatments for a range of entomological pests, including the insect orders Coleoptera, Diptera, Orthoptera, Hemiptera, and Lepidoptera [11–13].

2. History of EPN

The first entomopathogenic nematode (EPN) was initially described by Steiner in 1923 as *Aplectana kraussei*, which is now classified as *Steinernema kraussei*. In 1929, Steiner also introduced *Neoaplectana glaseri*, the first EPN species to be utilized for biological control, specifically targeting white grubs. In 1955, a nematode species, *Neoaplectana carpocapsae*, was identified by Weiser from the larvae of the codling moth (*Carpocapsa pomonella*). Interestingly, Dutky and Hough independently discovered the same species in the same host during the same year, with the isolate being designated as DD-136 for use in pest control. *Heterorhabditis bacteriophora* was first described by Pionar in 1976. Later, in 1994, Nguyen and Smart proposed the genus *Neosteinernema*, containing the species *N. longicurvicauda*. The most widely studied and utilized EPN species are found within the genera *Steinernema* and *Heterorhabditis*, which encompass the most significant species for biological control applications [14].

Entomopathogenic nematodes (EPNs) have developed the ability to detect and respond to plant-derived signals in order to locate potential herbivore hosts. When herbivores infest plant roots, they release a distinct set of molecules that differentiate them from healthy plants. The presence and spread of herbivore-induced plant volatiles (HIPVs) serve as a reliable indicator of herbivore activity. Additionally, EPNs utilize carbon dioxide, which is emitted by most living organisms, as a key cue for host location. This signal prompts foraging behavior in EPNs, with different life strategies such as ambushers and cruisers exhibiting varying levels of sensitivity to this stimulus. Furthermore, EPNs can exploit insect-specific chemical cues to locate their hosts more effectively. Herbivores continuously release various chemicals into the surrounding environment, including pheromones, exudates, molted skins (exuviae), and feces (frass). These insect-derived compounds, diffusing through the soil, can either attract or repel EPNs, or even induce behaviors such as nictation [15].

Heterorabditidae and *Steinernematide* are commonly used genera in pest management programs even though there are about 40 nematode families reported to control insect pests [16]. Around 100 species of *Steinernema* and 26 species of *Heterorhabditis* have been recorded worldwide [17, 18]. *Steinernema* and *Heterorhabditis* EPNs are known to be parasites of lepidopterans, coleopterans, and occasionally of orthopterans, dipterans, and hymenopterans [19–21].

Entomopathogenic nematodes (EPNs) employ two primary foraging strategies: ambushers and cruisers. Ambushers, such as *Steinernema carpocapsae*, adopt an energy-conserving approach, remaining stationary and waiting for mobile insect hosts to come within their reach, typically targeting pests in the upper soil layers like armyworms and cutworms. In contrast, cruisers are more active and typically subterranean, capable of traveling considerable distances to locate their host. These nematodes, including *Steinernema glaseri* and *Heterorhabditis bacteriophora*, are particularly effective against less mobile soil-dwelling pests, such as white grubs (Scarab beetles).

3. White trap method and multiplication

Infective juveniles (IJs) of entomopathogenic nematodes (EPNs) are commonly found in the soil and can be readily harvested by collecting samples from diverse environments such as agricultural fields, forests, riverbanks, pastures, and orchards across varying climatic conditions. Sampling is typically conducted using tools such as augers, tubes, shovels, and trowels. Two primary sampling techniques are generally used: stratified sampling and random sampling. Soil samples are typically collected from depths of up to 25 cm and from areas approximately 4 to 5 m^2 in size. A set of 3 to 5 sub-samples are taken per sample site and combined into a plastic bag for analysis. It is essential that the collected samples are clearly labeled with detailed information, including the location or site (preferably with GPS coordinates), the date of sampling, habitat type, prevailing vegetation, climatic conditions, altitude, and any insect pests observed at the sampling site.

The likelihood of naturally encountering EPN-infected insect cadavers in the field is relatively low, making insect baiting an essential and efficient method for isolating entomopathogenic nematodes (EPNs) from soil samples. Insect baiting is considered one of the simplest and most cost-effective approaches for attracting EPNs as well as insect pathogenic fungi [22]. In this technique, up to 100 grams of soil are placed in clean containers, and 4 to 5 *Galleria* larvae are introduced as bait. The containers are then sealed, inverted, and incubated in the dark at 25°C for 2 to 3 days, during which time mortality is monitored. Infected larvae exhibit distinct color changes: *Steinernema*-infected larvae turn yellow to brown, while *Heterorhabditis*-infected larvae turn red (**Figure 1A, B**). The cadavers are then carefully rinsed in sterile water and placed in white traps for the subsequent extraction of infective juveniles (IJs) and other developmental stages [24].

The white trap consists of a large dish (100 mm in diameter) containing a smaller petri dish (50 mm in diameter) lined with filter paper. Infected cadavers are placed on the smaller petri dish, and a small volume of sterile water is added. The setup is then incubated at 25°C. After 10 to 15 days, fresh infective juveniles (IJs) and other developmental stages can be collected from the suspension (**Figure 1C, D**). Entomopathogenic nematodes (EPNs) can be effectively cultured through both *in vitro* and *in vivo* methods under laboratory conditions. *In vivo* methods require living, susceptible insect hosts from orders such as Coleoptera, Lepidoptera, and Diptera to support the maintenance, growth, and reproduction of EPNs. In the absence of suitable insect hosts, the *in vitro* approach can be employed for rearing EPNs. The *in vitro* method involves the use of various media, including Nutrient Bromothymol Blue Agar (NBTA), liver-kidney agar, and lipid agar media, to provide essential nutrients to the nematodes and their symbiotic bacteria [25].

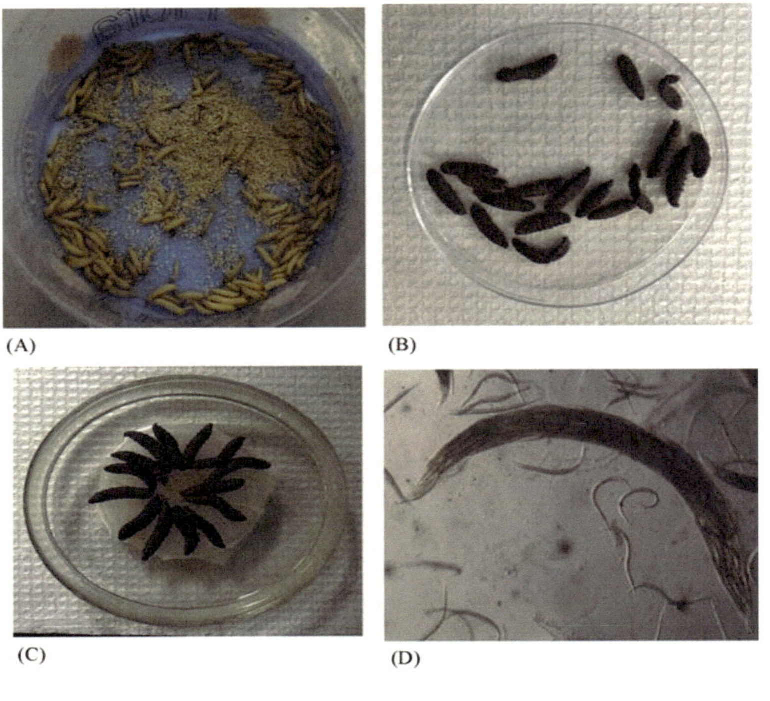

Figure 1.
Methodology for mass multiplication of Entomopathogenic nematode. Cadavers with body turned to a yellow to brown color indicate infection with Steinernematids, *while those that become red are infected by* Heterorhabditids *(A, B). The deceased cadavers are placed on the small petri dish, a small amount of sterile water is added, Fresh IJs and other developmental stages can be collected from the suspensions after a duration of 10 to 15 days (C, D) [4]. (Source: Singh et al. [23]).*

3.1 Relationship between bacterium and nematode

Entomopathogenic nematodes (EPNs) and their symbiotic bacteria engage in a mutualistic relationship, with each benefiting from the other. The nematode depends on the bacterium to kill its insect host, create a favorable environment for its development by producing antibiotics that inhibit competing microorganisms, and break down host tissues into nutrients. In return, the bacterium relies on the nematode for protection from external environmental threats, for facilitating penetration into the host's hemocoel, and for inhibiting the host's antibacterial defenses. This mutualistic association exhibits a high level of species specificity between the nematode and its bacterial partner [14]. It is well-documented that EPNs are naturally present in a variety of agro-ecosystems. However, direct observation of insect cadavers infected with EPNs is challenging, and the patchy distribution of infective juveniles (IJs) in soil often prevents their detection using standard nematode extraction methods (**Figure 2**) [26].

3.2 Multiplication of EPN

In vivo and *in vitro* methods are commonly employed for large-scale production of entomopathogenic nematodes (EPNs) [27]. However, *in vitro* mass production requires significant capital investment and specialized technical expertise. For a biological agent to be deemed successful, it is crucial that the host insect can be reared at a cost-effective rate and that the resulting product has a reasonably long shelf life. In contrast, although *in vivo* production of biocontrol agents necessitates lower financial investment and less technical expertise, scaling up the production process remains challenging, thereby making economic viability difficult to achieve [28]. Traditionally, *in vivo* mass rearing of EPNs has been conducted using the White trap method, initially developed by White in 1927 and subsequently modified [29]. Initially, the Baermann apparatus was used to recover infective juveniles (IJs) from cultures. Later, a novel method and apparatus were developed to harvest nematodes

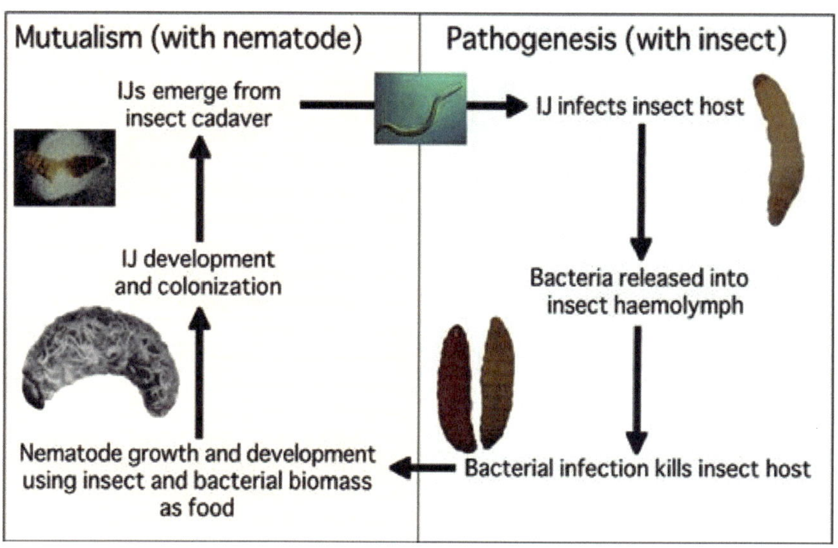

Figure 2.
The life cycle of Photorhabdus and Xenorhabdus [26].

from a mixture of charcoal and fecal samples, based on the migratory behavior of parasitic nematodes in their third larval stage (**Figure 3**) [30].

3.3 Isolation of symbiotic bacteria

Symbiotic bacteria were isolated from infected cadavers. Infected larva is surface sterilized by dipping into 95% ethanol. Larva is cut open with sterile forceps, and the hemolymph is streaked on Macconkey agar plates. Primary phase colonies appeared in red, bright pink color, while secondary phase colonies ranged from light yellow to brown color.

3.4 Solid media

Foam pieces of about 1 cm cubic size are used to enhance the surface area and aeration in the system. The foam pieces are impregnated with the bacteriological medium

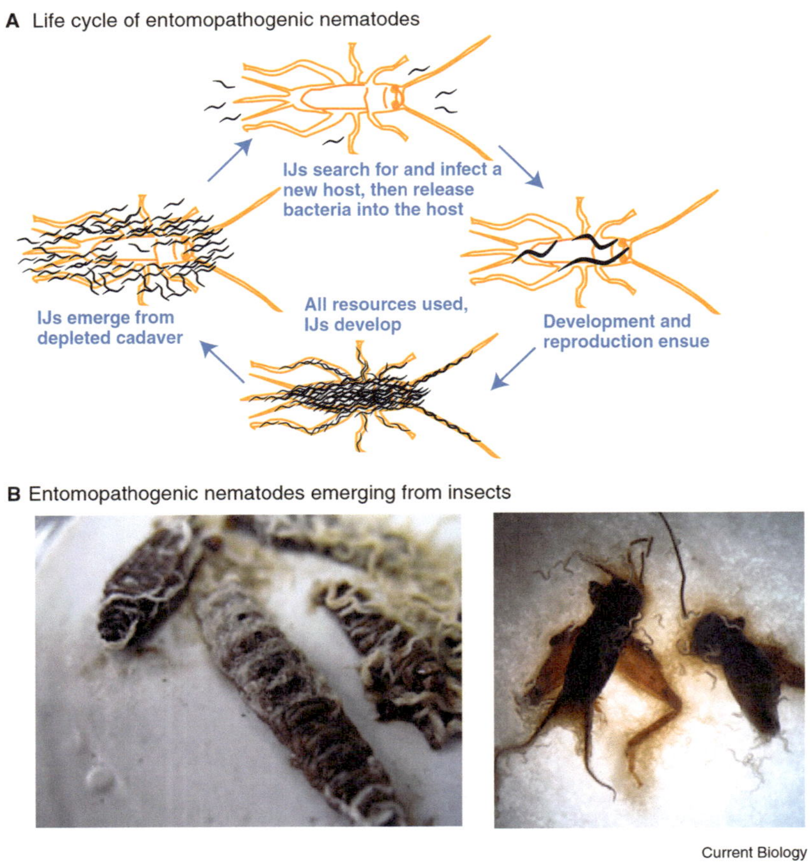
A Life cycle of entomopathogenic nematodes
IJs search for and infect a new host, then release bacteria into the host
Development and reproduction ensue
All resources used, IJs develop
IJs emerge from depleted cadaver
B Entomopathogenic nematodes emerging from insects
Current Biology

Figure 3.
(A) The infective juvenile (IJ) stage of the nematode seeks out a suitable host for infection by penetrating the host's hemolymph and releasing the pathogenic bacteria it carries. Within the insect host, the nematodes undergo development and reproduction, with multiple reproductive cycles occurring depending on the host's size. As the host's resources become depleted, a new generation of infective juveniles is produced, which then emerge and actively seek out new hosts to infect with the pathogenic bacteria. (B) Photographs depicting the emergence of entomopathogenic infective juveniles from Galleria mellonella *(waxworm larvae) on the left and* Acheta domestica *(crickets) on the right [30].*

(Wout's medium) and packed in 500 ml Erlenmeyer flasks before autoclaving. The bacteria are inoculated onto the foam pieces and allowed to attain proper stage for nematode inoculation. Pure culture of appropriate EPN strain is inoculated on the foam pieces. Such systems were optimized for large-scale production using large autoclavable plastic bags, and the first commercial production of EPNs was based on this system.

3.5 Liquid media

Commercial-level EPN production has to employ liquid culture systems involving fermentation technology. In this system, provision of adequate levels of oxygen and removal of carbon dioxide and other waste gaseous material must be regulated so that it does not damage the delicate, relatively large, reproducing EPNs or interfere with copulation [14]. The *in vitro* liquid culture of entomopathogenic nematodes (EPNs) begins in Erlenmeyer shake flasks, which provide necessary aeration and agitation. Following the initial phase of liquid culture, the process is scaled up to 5–20 L desktop bioreactors and subsequently to industrial-scale bioreactors ranging from 80 to 1000 L (**Figure 4**) [31].

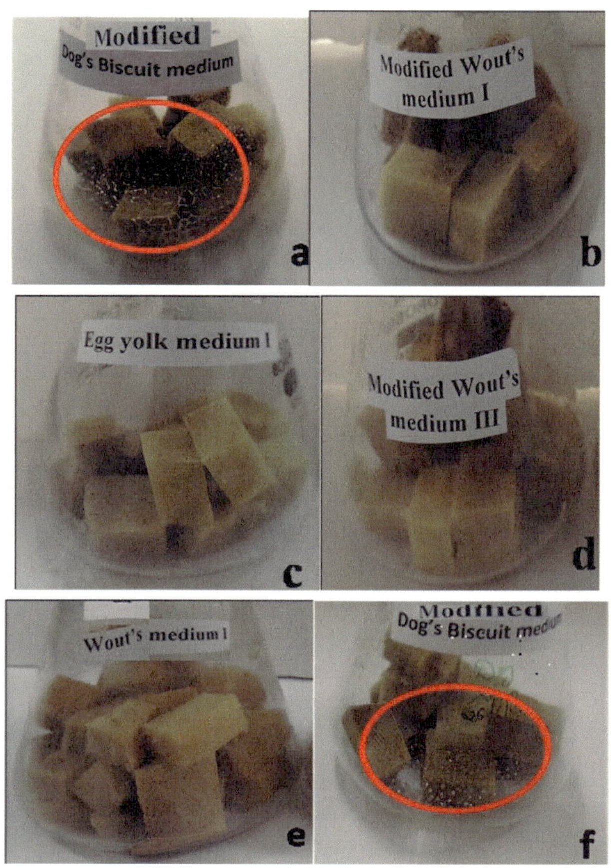

Figure 4.
Mass production of Entomopathogenic nematodes in different solid media: Multiplication of Heterorhabditis indica *after 30 days of nematode inoculation on: (a) Modified dog biscuit medium; (b) modified Wout's medium I; (c) modified Wout's medium III; (d) Wout's medium; and (e) multiplication of* Heterorhabditis indica *after 60 days of nematode inoculation on modified dog biscuit medium [31].*

In the cultivation of monoxenic liquid cultures of the bacto-helminthic complex, the production medium, comprising essential nutrients, chicken tissue, and lipids, was adjusted to physiological pH and pre-inoculated with a 5% culture of *Pseudomonas luminescens*. This culture was a 24-hour growth maintained at 28°C and 150 rpm in 2× nutrient broth (NB). The inoculation process was conducted in Sartorius Stedim Biostat bioreactors, specifically A+ with capacities of 2 and 5 L, and B+ with a 10 L capacity, with respective working volumes of 1.5, 4, and 7 L. The bioreactors were operated under the following conditions: a temperature of 28°C, agitation at 200 rpm, a pH of 7.30, and dissolved oxygen at 30%. Concurrently, nematodes were surface sanitized using a 0.125% Hyamine solution and subsequently rinsed with sterile tap water to eliminate residual Hyamine. Upon reaching the early stationary phase of bacterial growth (20–24 hours), the bioreactors were inoculated with the sanitized nematodes at a density of approximately 2000 infective juveniles (IJs)/mL, and cultivation continued at 28°C with a pH of 7.3. During the initial phase of bacterial growth, agitation was maintained at 200 rpm across all bioreactors, after which it was reduced to 100 rpm in bioreactor A+ and to 150 and 200 rpm in bioreactor B+, respectively. Following nematode inoculation, dissolved oxygen levels were sustained at 30% during bacterial growth and increased to 40% for nematode mass production. The bioreactors were operated in batch mode for a duration of 7–8 days [32].

4. Formulations

Nematodes intended for long-term storage and transportation to field sites can be formulated using various techniques. The formulation process should be carried out when the nematodes are fully active, either in motion or slightly desiccated, to reduce their mobility [33]. Since entomopathogenic nematodes (EPNs) are live, multicellular organisms, their quality tends to deteriorate over time, regardless of the formulation method, due to the depletion of their internal reserves. This decline is primarily attributed to the consumption of lipid reserves by the nematodes [34]. Two primary strategies are utilized to improve the suitability of formulations for the storage and transportation of nematodes. The first strategy involves the use of inert carriers, such as sponge or vermiculite, which ensure sufficient gaseous exchange. The second strategy is the induction of partial anhydrobiosis, a process that reduces the metabolic activity of the nematodes, thereby conserving their energy reserves [35].

4.1 Advantages of EPN

- High host search ability.
- Compatible with pesticides and other biocontrol agents of insect pests.
- Capability of causing mortality of insects within 48–72 hours after infection.
- Ability for mass multiplication on artificial media.
- EPNs are viable for up to 3–6 months when refrigerated at 4 to 10°C.
- EPNs can be easily applied in field using conventional sprayers and do not require any special equipment.

- EPNs are safe for humans, vertebrates, and non-target organisms.
- EPNs are exempt from registration requirements in many countries.

4.2 Disadvantages of EPN

- Intolerance or mortality of the free-living stages of nematodes to low humidity and extreme temperatures.
- Nematodes need to be protected from ultraviolet light, which soon reduces the infectivity and may kill the infective stages.
- The relatively slow rate at which microorganisms kill their hosts, compared to chemical insecticides, has hindered their effectiveness and limited their acceptance among potential users.

5. Efficacy of EPN against various insect pests

5.1 Efficacy of EPN against lepidopteran pests

The single-concentration screening assay revealed that, out of 10 entomopathogenic nematode (EPN) isolates tested, *Heterorhabditis indica* 1NBAIIH38, *H. indica* 2NBAIIH03, *H. bacteriophora* NBAIRH75, *Steinernema carpocapsae* NBAIRS59, and *S. siamkayai* 3 NBAIIS31 caused more than 50% mortality in 3rd instar larvae of *Spodoptera frugiperda*. Among these, *H. indica* 1NBAIIH38 exhibited the highest mortality (78%), while *S. abbasi* 2 NBAIIS49 caused the lowest mortality (20%). Further analysis indicated a significant variation in virulence among the EPN isolates, highlighting the importance of selecting the most virulent isolates for effective management of target insect pests [36].

Experiments conducted using the entomopathogenic nematode (EPN) *Heterorhabditis indica* (isolate: CICR Guava) on filter paper demonstrated its efficacy against *Galleria mellonella* and *Spodoptera litura*. The results indicated that *H. indica* caused 100% mortality in 5th instar larvae of *G. mellonella* at a treatment dose of 40 infective juveniles (IJs)/100 μl within 72 hours of infection. For S. *litura*, 100% mortality was recorded within 72 hours at a treatment dose of 100 IJs/100 μl in 3rd instar larvae, which exhibited higher susceptibility. These findings suggest a positive correlation between the concentration of nematode treatment, exposure time, and insect mortality in tobacco cutworm larvae. Thus, the *H. indica* isolate (CICR-Guava) can be recommended as a potential biocontrol agent for managing *S. litura* in the Vidarbha region [37]. The study also evaluated the susceptibility of *S. litura* to four locally isolated EPN species: *H. indica*, *Heterorhabditis baujardi*, *Steinernema sangi*, and *Steinernema surkhetense*. The LC50 values of *H. indica* at 72 hours post-incubation were 20.26 and 62.07 IJs/larva for the 3rd and 5th instars, respectively, and 913.34 IJs/pupa. The high mortality caused by *H. indica* and *H. baujardi* may be attributed to their high rate of penetration, typical of Heterorhabditids [38]. However, despite a lower penetration rate, *S. sangi* exhibited a similar level of pathogenicity to the Heterorhabditids. In laboratory bioassays comparing the biocontrol potential of *Steinernema siamkayai* (IIVR JNC01) with the commercially available *H. indica* (NBAIIH38 strain) against 3rd instar larvae of *S. litura*, *Spilosoma obliqua*, and

Spoladea recurvalis, *S. siamkayai* (IIVR JNC01) caused 100, 100, and 85% mortality in these larvae, respectively [39].

The exploration and identification of native EPN species and strains adapted to local agro-climatic conditions is a crucial step in developing biocontrol agents for integrated pest management programs targeting major insect pests..The efficacy of eight native entomopathogenic nematodes (EPNs) against larvae of the hairy caterpillar (*Euproctis* sp.) and the shoot borer (*Conogethes punctiferalis*) was evaluated. Among the tested EPN isolates, all except *Oscheius* sp. IISR 08 caused 100% mortality in the larvae of the hairy caterpillar. *Heterorhabditis* sp. (IISR 01), *Steinernema* sp. (IISR 02), and *Oscheius* sp. (IISR 07 and 08) also caused 100% mortality in the larvae of the shoot borer [40].

5.2 Efficacy of EPN against hemipteran pests

The efficacy of native entomopathogenic nematodes (EPNs) against *Planococcus citri* was evaluated under laboratory conditions at various concentrations (80, 100, 150, 200 IJs/adult) and temperatures (20, 25, 30°C). The highest efficacy (68%) was achieved by *Heterorhabditis indica* 216-H at the highest concentration (200 IJs) at 25°C. Mortality rates were generally higher at 25°C compared to the other temperatures tested, and *H. indica* 216-H outperformed other EPN species at this temperature across all concentrations. These results suggest that *H. indica* 216-H holds significant potential for the control of *P. citri* [41]. In a separate study, the efficacy of *Steinernema feltiae* and *H. bacteriophora* against *Dactylopius opuntiae* was assessed. The results indicated that *S. feltiae* was more effective, causing a mortality rate of 98.8% in nymphs after 8 days of exposure, while *H. bacteriophora* resulted in a lower mortality rate of 83.8% [42].

5.3 Efficacy of EPN against coleopteran pests

S. siamkayai (IIVR JNC01 strain) caused 92.5% mortality of 2nd instar grubs of *Myllocerus subfasciatus* under laboratory conditions [39]. The bioefficacy of *S. dharanaii* (TFRIEPN-15) against white grub, *Holotrichia rustica* revealed that the minimum number of IJs, i.e., 300 Grub^{-1}, causes 13.33% mortality in younger 6 days after the exposure, followed by 46.66% at the IJs population of 600 IJs Grub^{-1} [43]. The investigation on bioefficacy of entomopathogenic nematode, *H. indica* against white grub noted that mortality of white grub reached up to 73.34% at higher inoculums level (100 IJs/grub) after 120 hrs of application [44]. The study on the mortality of *Capnodis tenebrionis* larvae caused by different EPNs at different days after application exposed that after 1 D, larval mortality was 62.5, 52.5, 70.0, 50.0, and 0.00% with *S. feltiae, S. carpocapsae, S. affine, H. bacteriophora,* and control, respectively [45]. The efficacy of *H. indica* (DSM78) against naturally infested sugarcane white grub (*H. serrata*) was experimented under field conditions. The reduction in grub population due to EPN treatment ranged between 43.5 and 77% at field trial I and 30–78% at field trial II [46]. The bioefficacy of entomopathogenic nematodes against the white grub (*Anomala communis*) in potato was evaluated under field conditions. The highest larval mortality was observed 96 hours after treatment with *Steinernema glaseri* at a rate of 5 × 10^9 infective juveniles (IJs)/ha, followed by *S. glaseri* at 2.5 × 10^9 IJs/ha. The highest grub mortality (58.32%) was recorded with *S. glaseri* at 5 × 10^9 IJs/

ha. Additionally, tuber damage was reduced to 24.99%, and the increase in yield was 15.78 t/ha when treated with *S. glaseri* at 5 × 10^9 IJs/ha [47].

5.4 Efficacy of EPN against dipteran pests

The experiments on the mortality of *Bactrocera zonata* and *Bactrocera dorsalis* adults when exposed to ten different species of entomopathogenic nematodes in Petri plates expressed that at all periods (12, 24, 48, and 72 h) and for both fly species, *H. bacteriophora* caused higher mortality than all other EPN species except *S. carpocapsae* [48].

5.5 Compatibility of EPN with insecticides

The compatibility of the entomopathogenic nematode *Heterorhabditis indica* with seven insecticides registered by the Central Insecticide Board was assessed under laboratory conditions. The results indicated that *H. indica* was most compatible with imidacloprid 17.8SL, as the highest percentage of live nematodes was observed 72 hours after exposure to this insecticide. *H. indica* also demonstrated compatibility with fipronil 5SC up to 48 hours of exposure. In contrast, less than 70% of *H. indica* remained viable after exposure to thiamethoxam 25WG, diafenthiuron 50WP, and cypermethrin 25EC, indicating that these insecticides were least compatible with the nematodes. Additionally, emamectin benzoate 5SG and chlorpyrifos 20EC were found to be incompatible with *H. indica* after 48 hours of exposure [49].

In laboratory bioassays, both *S. carpocapsae* and *H. bacteriophora* exhibited high tolerance to azadirachtin- and neonicotinoid-based insecticides, with survival rates ranging from 96.1 to 99.7 percent after 72 hours of exposure. *S. carpocapsae* demonstrated significantly higher virulence against last instar larvae of *Agrotis ipsilon* than *H. bacteriophora* at all tested concentrations. Larval mortality increased with both nematode concentration and exposure duration. At 160 infective juveniles (IJs) per larva, *S. carpocapsae* achieved cent percent mortality, while *H. bacteriophora* reached 90 per-cent after 72 hours. Combined applications of EPNs (80 IJs/larva) with either azadirachtin or neonicotinoid insecticides significantly enhanced larval mortality compared to individual treatments. Among combinations, EPNs with azadirachtin were more effective than those with neonicotinoids [50].

5.6 Compatibility of EPN with entomopathogenic fungi

The laboratory assays, *Beauveria bassiana*, *Metarhizium anisopliae*, and *H. bacteriophora,* showed significant pathogenicity against larval instars of *Rhynchophorus ferrugineus*. Synergistic effects were more frequent in *H. bacteriophora* + *B. bassiana* combinations, particularly in second and fourth instars at 0, 7, and 14 days, and in sixth instars at 0 and 7 days. Combined treatments reduced pupation, adult emergence, and egg hatching more than individual applications. Sub-lethal doses led to decreased larval weight, food consumption, frass production, and altered development. The *H. bacteriophora* + *B. bassiana* combination consistently showed the highest efficacy, especially against early instars [51].

Laboratory screening of EPNs for infectivity can be an important step in developing a biological control programme for a particular pest [52]. One of the main reasons for failure of EPNs as biological control of insect pests is the wrong choice of nematode species or strain [53] as results can vary greatly even among strains of the same species.

6. Conclusions

Entomopathogenic nematodes (EPNs) have emerged as highly promising biological control agents for insect pest management, owing to their numerous attributes that align with the key characteristics of ideal biocontrol agents. These nematodes can be efficiently cultivated both in controlled laboratory conditions (*in vitro*) and within their natural environments (*in vivo*). Various types of insect pests that inhabit foliage and soil, such as coleopteran (white grub), dipteran (leaf miner), and lepidopteran (hairy caterpillar), can be effectively managed through the application of EPNs. What sets these nematodes apart is their compatibility with other crucial elements of Integrated Pest Management (IPM), including various chemical insecticides and other biological pesticides. This compatibility enhances their efficacy and versatility within integrated pest management strategies. The potential for developing and utilizing entomopathogenic nematodes as a sustainable option for pest control is substantial, highlighting their importance as a key component of environmentally friendly and holistic pest management.

7. Future thrust

Future research and development should focus on advancing the practical applications of entomopathogenic nematodes (EPNs) in diverse agricultural systems. Efforts should aim to improve mass production techniques to make EPNs more cost-effective and accessible for large-scale use. Additionally, further studies on their compatibility with advanced Integrated Pest Management (IPM) tools, including novel formulations of biopesticides and precision agriculture technologies, will help maximize their effectiveness. Exploration of their potential in managing emerging pest threats and adapting to varying climatic conditions is also crucial. By leveraging innovative delivery systems and fostering collaborations between researchers, policymakers, and farmers, the full potential of EPNs as sustainable and environmentally sound pest control agents can be fully realized.

Conflict of interest

The authors declare no conflict of interest.

Author details

Thattankandy Meethal Aparna, Mukesh R. Siddhapara* and Sonam Kumari
Department of Entomology, Navsari Agricultural University, Navsari, Gujarat, India

*Address all correspondence to: agrilmak@nau.in

References

[1] Chakraborty N, Mitra R, Pal S, Ganguly R, Acharya K, Minkina T, et al. Biopesticide consumption in India: Insights into the current trends. Agriculture. 2023;**13**(3):557. DOI: 10.3390/agriculture13030557

[2] Central Insecticides Board and Registration Committee. Bio-Pesticide Registrant. Faridabad: Directorate of Plant Protection Quarantine & Storage, Department of Agriculture and Farmers Welfare, Government of India; 2025. Available from: https://ppqs.gov.in/divisions/cib-rc/bio-pesticide-registrant [Accessed: March 28, 2025]

[3] Yadav R. Biopesticides: Current status and future prospects. Proceedings of the International Academy of Ecology and Environmental Sciences. 2022;**12**(3):211

[4] US Environmental Protection Agency (US EPA). Health Effects of Ozone Pollution. Washington DC: US Environmental Protection Agency (US EPA); 2022. Available from: https://www.epa.gov/ground-level-ozone-pollution/health-effects-ozone-pollution [Accessed: March 28, 2025]

[5] Curl CL, Spivak M, Phinney R, Montrose L. Synthetic pesticides and health in vulnerable populations: Agricultural workers. Current Environmental Health Reports. 2020;**7**:13-29. DOI: 10.1007/s40572-020-00266-5

[6] Shah R. Pesticides and human health [Internet]. In: Emerging Contaminants. London, UK: IntechOpen; 2021. DOI: 10.5772/intechopen.93806

[7] Drugmand D, Feit S, Fuhr L, Muffett C. Fossils, Fertilizers, and False Solutions: How Laundering Fossil Fuels in Agrochemicals Puts the Climate and the Planet at Risk. Washington, DC: Center for International Environmental Law; 2022

[8] Lacey LA, Georgis R. Entomopathogenic nematodes for control of insect pests above and below ground with comments on commercial production. Journal of Nematology. 2012;**44**:218-225

[9] Gaugler R. Entomopathogenic Nematodes in Biological Control. 1st ed. CRC Press; 1990. DOI: 10.1201/9781351071741

[10] Glazer I. Survival and efficacy of Steinernema carpocapsae in an exposed environment. Biocontrol Science and Technology. 1992;**2**(2):101-107

[11] Hatting JL, Moore SD, Malan AP. Microbial control of phytophagous invertebrate pests in South Africa: Current status and future prospects. Journal of Invertebrate Pathology. 2019;**165**:54-66

[12] Sharma MP, Sharma AN, Hussaini SS. Entomopathogenic nematodes, a potential microbial biopesticide: Mass production and commercialisation status – A mini review. Archives of Phytopathology and Plant Protection. 2011;**44**:855-870

[13] Labaude S, Griffin CT. Transmission success of entomopathogenic nematodes used in pest control. Insects. 2018;**9**(2):72. DOI: 10.3390/insects9020072

[14] Walia RK, Bajaj HK. Text Book on Introductory Plant Nematology. 2nd rev ed. New Delhi: ICAR; 2014. p. 240

[15] Zhang XL, Kesner L, Robert CAM. Chemical host-seeking cues of entomopathogenic nematodes. Current Opinion in Insect Science. 2021;**44**:72-81

[16] Kaya HK, Koppenhofer AM. Biological control of insects and other invertebrates with nematodes. In: Chen ZX, Chen SY, Dickson DW, editors. Nematology, Advances and Perspectives. Wallingford: CAB Int; 2004. pp. 1083-1132

[17] Cimen H, Puza V, Nermut J, Hatting J, Ramakuwela T, Hazir S. Steinernema biddulphin sp., a new entomopathogenic nematode (Nematoda: Steinernematidae) from South Africa. Journal of Nematology. 2016;**48**:148-158

[18] Shahina F, Tabassum KA, Salma J, Mehreen G, Knoetze R. Heterorhabditis pakistanensis sp. (Nematoda: Heterorhabditidae), a new entomopathogenic nematode from Pakistan. Journal of Helminthology. 2016;**4**:1-4. DOI: 10.1017/S0022149×16000158

[19] Klein MG. Efficacy against soil inhabiting insect pests. In: Gaugler R, Kaya HK, editors. Entomopathogenic Nematodes in Biological Control. Boca Raton: CRC Press; 1990. pp. 195-214. DOI: 10.1201/9781351071741-14

[20] Poinar GO Jr. Taxonomy and biology of Steinermematidae and Heterorhabditidae. In: Gaugler R, Kaya HK, editors. Entomopathogenic Nematodes in Biological Control. Boca Raton: CRC Press; 1990. pp. 23-61. DOI: 10.1007/978-3-030-26657-8_11

[21] Grewal PS, Ehlers RU, Shapiro-Ilan DI. Nematodes as Biocontrol Agents. Wallingford: CABI Publishing; 2005. DOI: 10.1079/9780851990170.0000

[22] Bedding RA, Akhurst RJ. A simple technique for the detection of insect parasitic rhabditid nematodes in soil. Nematologica. 1975;**21**:109-110

[23] Singh AK, Kumar M, Ahuja A, Vinay BK, Kommu KK, Thakur S, et al. Entomopathogenic nematodes: A sustainable option for insect pest management. In: Gul H, editor. Biopesticides. 1st ed. Amsterdam: Elsevier; 2022. pp. 73-92. DOI: 10.1016/B978-0-12-823355-9.00007-9

[24] White GF. A method for obtaining infective nematode larvae from cultures. Science. 1927;**66**:302. DOI: 10.1126/science.66.1709.302-a

[25] McMullen JG, Stock SP. In vivo and in vitro rearing of entomopathogenic nematodes (*Steinernematidae* and *Heterorhabditidae*). Journal of Visualized Experiments. 2014;**91**:e52096

[26] Goodrich-Blair H, Clarke DJ. Mutualism and pathogenesis in Xenorhabdus and Photorhabdus: Two roads to the same destination. Molecular Microbiology. 2007;**64**(2):260-268

[27] Gaugler R, Han R. Production technology. In: Gaugler R, editor. Entomopathogenic Nematology. New York: CABI; 2002. pp. 289-310

[28] Shapiro-Ilan DI, Gaugler R. Production technology for entomopathogenic nematodes and their bacterial symbionts. Journal of Industrial Microbiology & Biotechnology. 2002;**28**:137-146. DOI: 10.1038/sj/jim/7000230

[29] Dutky SR, Thompson JV, Cantwell GE. A technique for the mass propagation of the DD-136 nematode. Journal of Invertebrate Pathology. 1964;**6**:417-422

[30] Dillman AR, Sternberg PW. Entomopathogenic nematodes. Current Biology. 2012;**22**(11):R430-R431

[31] Kranti KVVS, Kumar GN. Mass multiplication of entomopathogenic nematodes on *in vitro* solid media. International Journal of Current Microbiology and Applied Sciences. 2018;**7**(7):3282-3292

[32] Upadhyay D, Mandjiny S, Bullard-Dillard R, Storms M, Menefee M, Holmes LD. Lab-scale in vitro mass production of the entomopathogenic nematode *Heterorhabditis bacteriophora* using liquid culture fermentation technology. American Journal of Bioscience and Bioengineering. 2015;**3**(6):203-207

[33] Grewal PS. Formulation and application technology. In: Gaugler R, editor. Entomopathogenic Nematology. Wallingford: CABI Publishing; 2002. pp. 265-287. DOI: 10.1079/9780851995670.0265

[34] Lewis EE, Perez EE. Formulation and storage of entomopathogenic nematodes. International Journal of Nematology. 2004;**14**:30-34

[35] Grewal PS, Peters A. Formulation and quality. In: Grewal PS, Ehlers RU, Shapiro-Ilan DI, editors. Nematodes as Biocontrol Agents. Wallingford: CABI International; 2005. pp. 79-90

[36] Patil J, Linga V, Vijayakumar R, Subaharan K, Navik O, Bakthavatsalam N, et al. Biocontrol potential of entomopathogenic nematodes for the sustainable management of Spodoptera frugiperda in maize. Pest Management Science. 2022;**78**(7):2883-2895

[37] Supriya K, Dash SS, Ingole DB, Kashyap DP, Lavhe NV, Tambe VJ. Evaluationofentomopathogenicnematode (EPN) isolate, *Heterorhabditis indica* of Vidarbha region, against the tobacco cutworm, *Spodoptera litura*. Environment Conservation Journal. 2022;**23**(3):35-41

[38] Lalramnghaki HC, Lalramliana LHT, Vanlalhlimpuia LM, Vanramliana. Susceptibility of the fall armyworm, Spodoptera frugiperda, to four species of entomopathogenic nematodes. Egyptian Journal of Biological Pest Control. 2021;**31**:1-11

[39] Gowda MT, Patil J, Halder J, Veereshkumar DPA, Rai AB, et al. Isolation, identification and biocontrol potential of entomopathogenic nematodes in Purvanchal and Bundelkhand regions of Uttar Pradesh. Egyptian Journal of Biological Pest Control. 2020;**30**:1-11

[40] Pervez R, Eapen SJ, Devasahayam S, Jacob TK. Efficacy of some entomopathogenic nematodes against insect pests of ginger and their multiplication. Nematologia Mediterranea. 2012;**40**:39-44

[41] Najm ES, Yuksel E, Canhilal R. Biocontrol potential of Turkish entomopathogenic nematodes against the citrus mealybug *Planococcus citri*. KSUT Tarım Doga Derg. 2023;**26**(1):55-61

[42] El A, Mokrini M, Dababat F, Lahlali RA, Sbaghi M. Moroccan entomopathogenic nematodes as biocontrol agents against *Dactylopius opuntiae*. Scientific Reports. 2022;**12**(1):75-90

[43] Paunikar SD, Kulkarni N. Bioefficacy of new species of entomopathogenic nematode Steinernema dharanaii against whitegrub Holotrichia rustica. International Journal of Advancement in Life Sciences Research. 2020;**3**(3):20-29

[44] Kamaliya RP, Jethva DM, Kachhadiya NM, Ahir VR, Vala GS. Bio-efficacy of Heterorhabditis indica against groundnut white grub. International Journal of Current Microbiology and Applied Sciences. 2019;**8**(4):830-836

[45] Sahin C, Gozel U. Efficacy of entomopathogenic nematodes against neonate larvae of *Capnodis tenebrionis*. Turkish Journal of Entomology. 2019;**43**(3):279-285

[46] Sankaranarayanan C, Singaravelu B, Rajeshkumar M. Entomopathogenic nematodes (EPN): Diversity in Indian tropical sugarcane ecosystem and biocontrol potential against white grub *Holotrichia serrata*. Sugar Tech. 2019;**21**:371-382

[47] Sharmila R, Subramanian S, Poornima K, Anitha K. Biocontrol efficacy of entomopathogenic nematodes on white grubs, Anomala communis, in potato. International Journal of Research Studies in Zoology. 2019;**5**(4):8-15

[48] Usman M, Wakil W, Shapiro-Ilan DI. Entomopathogenic nematodes as biological control agents against *Bactrocera zonata* and *B. dorsalis*. Biological Control. 2021;**163**:104706

[49] Dash SS, Koosari S, Ingole DB, Kashyap DP, Tambe VJ, Lavhe NV. Compatibility studies of *Heterorhabditis indica* with newer insecticides under lab conditions. Environment Conservation Journal. 2022;**23**(3):42-46

[50] Mahmoud MF, Mahfouz HM, KM M. Compatibility of entomopathogenic nematodes with neonicotinoids and azadirachtin for controlling *Agrotis ipsilon* in canola. International Journal of Environmental Sciences. 2016;**2**(1):11-18

[51] Wakil W, Yasin M, Shapiro-Ilan D. Effects of single and combined applications of fungi and nematodes against Rhynchophorus ferrugineus. Scientific Reports. 2017;**7**(1):59-71

[52] Ricci M, Glazer I, Gaugler R. Entomopathogenic nematodes infectivity assay: Comparison of laboratory bioassay. Biocontrol Science and Technology. 1996;**6**:235-245

[53] Georgis R, Gaugler R. Predictability in biological control using entomopathogenic nematodes. Journal of Economic Entomology. 1991;**84**:713-720

Chapter 3

Phytoparasitic Nematodes Affecting Kyrgyzstan's Vegetable Crops and Examining the Predatory Fungus *Arthrobotrys oligospora* as a Biological Control Agent

Tinatin Doolotkeldieva

Abstract

Parasitic nematodes are some of the most harmful plant pathogens, and their detrimental impact on crops is increasing in Kyrgyzstan. Notably, the potato stem nematode (*Ditylenchus destructor*) and the stalk garlic nematode (*Ditylenchus dipsaci*) threaten economically essential crops such as potatoes, garlic, sugar beets, and rice. Losses for these crops exceed 50% of the total harvest. Chemical nematicides are used in large quantities to fight them, but the high risk of environmental pollution leads to the search for an alternative way. Predatory fungi that create specialized traps and use nematodes as food are particularly valuable. *Arthrobotry's oligospora Fres (Orbiliomycetes)* is the best-known species that performs this function as an active biological agent in the fight against parasitic nematodes. This study aimed to isolate and identify predatory fungi from various natural objects using classical mycology alongside modern molecular methods. In vitro and in vivo screening of potential predatory fungal isolates was conducted to select highly effective strains for the control of parasitic nematodes. A total of 12 natural isolates of *Arthrobotrys oligospora* were assessed for their predatory efficacy against garlic and potato stem nematodes.

Keywords: potato nematode, garlic nematode, nematophagous fungi, *Arthrobotrys oligospora*, biological control

1. Introduction

Among the most dangerous plant pathogens are phytohelminths, parasitic nematodes that significantly reduce the yield and quality of several important crops. These soil pathogens are especially harmful in intensive farming conditions. For certain crops, such as sugar beets and potatoes, losses can often exceed 50% of the total harvest. Research on the phytohelminth fauna affecting crops in Kyrgyzstan has been conducted over several years. This text offers a brief overview of those studies on these parasitic organisms.

1.1 The knowledge level and prevalence of plant-parasitic nematodes in the agroecological systems of Kyrgyzstan

According to a research by Dzhunusov [1], a group of soil-dwelling nematodes called devisaprobionts has been identified in wheat and barley. This group consists of 14 genera and 27 species. The most common genera in this group include *Acrobeles, Acrobeloides, Eucephalobus, Cephalobus, Chiloplacus,* and *Panagrolaimus.* Additionally, there are phytohelminths with non-specific pathogenic effects, encompassing seven genera and 16 species, with the most prevalent genera being *Tylenchus* and *Aphelenchus.* Groups of ectoparasitic mycohelminths, perforators, and phytohelminths with specific pathogenic effects are represented by 12 genera and 19 species. Notable genera in this category include *Aphelenchoides, Ditylenchus, Hrlicotylenchus, Tylenchorhynchus*, and *Pratylenchus.* In the sugar beet fields of the Chui Valley, researchers identified 14 species of parasitic nematodes belonging to eight different genera. The most commonly found species include *Pratylenchus crenatus, Pratylenchus pratensis, Paratylenchus nanus, Rotylenchus robustus, and Heterodera schachtii*. Notably, the sugar beet cyst nematode (*H. schachtii*) and the worm-like parasitic nematodes of *Pratylenchus* were present in all sugar beet cultivation areas throughout the Chui Valley [2].

In terms of ecological groups and the qualitative composition of nematodes associated with sugar beets grown in crop rotation, the distribution of individuals in both the root-soil and the root system of the sugar beet is as follows: pararhizobionts constitute 15.4% in the root-soil and 0% in the root system. *Deisaprobes* comprise 20.9% in the root-soil and 56.3% in the root system. *Eusaprobes* account for 21.3% of the root soil and 0.9% of the root system [3].

The dominant nematode species in potato plantings include *Aphelenchoides parietinus, Panagrolaimus rigidus*, and others. Among the true parasites, the root-knot nematode (*Meloidogine incognita*) and the potato stem nematode (*Ditylenchus dipsaci*) have been recorded in significant quantities in the soil and underground organs. The latter is responsible for plant helminthiasis in several surveyed farms in Kyrgyzstan's Issyk-Kul and Chui regions. The composition of nematodes found in vegetable crops in Kyrgyzstan was analyzed, focusing specifically on phytoparasitic species [1, 4, 5]. The most nematode species were identified in tomato, onion, and garlic plants, while the lowest was observed in pepper and cabbage. The dominant families across all plant organs and their rhizospheres were Cephalobidae, Panagrolaimidae, and Aphelenchidae. The most abundant species included *Panagrolaimus rigidus, Acrobeloides nanus, Cephalobus persegnia,* and *Ditylenchus intermedia.* Notably, the phytoparasite *Pratylenchus pratensis* was found to affect the roots of cabbage, onion, and garlic plants. Additionally, species from the Ditylenchus and Helicotylenchus genera were detected in the roots and root-soil of cabbage, pepper, and tomato plants [5].

In the parasitic nematode fauna associated with alfalfa, over 50 species from 15 genera have been identified. However, only a few of these are causative agents of nematode diseases. The main nematodes responsible for such diseases include stem nematodes (*Ditylenchus* spp.), root-knot nematodes (*Meloidogyne* spp.), and short-bodied nematodes (*Pratylenchus* spp.) [6].

The nematode fauna complex associated with alfalfa phytohelminths comprises several genera, each with specific percentages identified in the root-soil and root systems. The genera and their respective percentages are as follows: - Pratylenchus: 6.4% in root-soil and 22.7% in root systems; Aphelenchus: 6.8% in root-soil and 4.8%

in root systems; Aphelenchoides: 2.9% in root-soil and 6.1% in root systems; Ditylenchus: 11.7% in root-soil and 3.5% in root systems; Tylenchus: 10.8% in root-soil and 11.4% in root systems; Helicotylenchus: 8.3% in root-soil and 4.5% in root systems; Tylenchorhynchus: 11.9% in root-soil and 2.9% in root systems [7].

The comparison of the frequency of individual genera of phytonematodes in fields with crop rotation versus those with permanent alfalfa cultivation revealed a notable contrast. In the crop rotation fields, 13 out of 29 detected genera were present in more than one-third of the samples. In contrast, in fields with permanent alfalfa cultivation, a significantly higher number of genera—18 out of 29—were found with the exact prevalence [7]. The presence of dangerous root parasites of the genus Pratylenchus in the examined crops is noteworthy. Additionally, many nematodes from *the Aphelenchoides* and *Aphelenchus* genera across all fields suggest that phytoparasitic fungi may be present in soil. The high proportion of the *Ditylenchus* genus is likely due to an outbreak of this disease in the studied crops and fields. It is well documented that *Ditylenchus dipsaci* has over 40 races and can affect a wide range of cultivated and weed plant species [7].

1.2 Biological traits and harmful effects of the stem nematode (*Ditylenchus dipsaci*) and tuber nematode (*Ditylenchus destructor*) in crops

The stem nematode, *Ditylenchus dipsaci*, is a type of roundworm (phytohelminth) that affects the underground parts of various plants. Approximately 450 races of this nematode infect around 450 plant species. *D. dipsaci* can infest important crops such as sugar beets, table beets, tomatoes, eggplants, carrots, onions, peppers, garlic, and various pumpkins, including cucumbers. It also impacts sunflowers, cereals, legumes, and hops and is found in various weeds. This nematode can infect ornamental crops and particularly damages potatoes [8]. *D. dipsaci* is a microscopic worm that measures approximately 1.5 mm in length. It can penetrate plants from the soil, through infected planting material, or sometimes from seeds. These worms inhabit the intercellular spaces of plants, particularly between the scales of onion and garlic bulbs. They feed on cell sap and can lay up to 250 eggs per season. Under optimal temperature conditions, ranging from 15 to 20°C, up to six generations can develop within a single season [9]. Research has identified the stem nematode *Ditylenchus dipsaci* as one of the many parasites affecting vegetable crops in Kyrgyzstan, particularly onions and garlic. This polyphagous plant-parasitic nematode is found worldwide and comprises over 20 biological races that primarily differ in their host plant preferences. In Kyrgyzstan, surveys indicate that *Ditylenchus dipsaci* is consistently present in nearly all areas where onions are cultivated intensively, especially in the Chui region. In areas with continuous onion farming, such as the Sokuluk and Moscow regions, damage from this nematode has been observed to range from 60 to 90%. Consequently, crop losses often amount to 15–25%, with total losses ranging from 58 to 77 quintals per hectare [5].

The tube nematode (Ditylenchus destructor) is a type of roundworm, a phytohelminth. It primarily affects the underground parts of plants. This nematode thrives in temperatures ranging from +5 to +34°C and can develop within 18 to 68 days. It typically overwinters at either the egg or fourth larval stage. In recent years, damage to potato tubers caused by stem nematodes has been recorded annually. The harm caused by these nematodes lies in their ability to damage tubers, leading to secondary infections. As a result, the tubers may rot or decline in their commercial and seed quality [10]. The potato stem nematode (Ditylenchus destructor) significantly reduces seed tuber quality and increases potato waste during storage. This situation underscores the need for collective action, as only 2 of the 12 farms surveyed in the Jety-Oguz and Ak-Suu districts of Issyk-Kul, as well as in the Alamedin, Sokuluk, and Moskovsky districts of the Chui region, were free of this nematode [1, 4].

1.3 Predatory fungi *Arthrobotrys oligospora* as a biological agent against soil parasitic nematodes

Annual cycles of plant nematode infestations result in a significant buildup of soil parasites, making effective, sustainable control crucial. While chemical methods using nematicides can be effective, they often harm the environment and non-parasitic soil organisms [11, 12]. Additionally, frequent use of anthelmintics can lead to parasite resistance, which may require higher doses or alternative products, further raising environmental concerns. This underscores the need to develop environmentally friendly control alternatives [13, 14]. Nematophagous fungi play a vital role in naturally controlling parasitic nematodes, offering an ecological solution to this issue. Approximately 200 fungal species can attack active nematodes. These fungi use unique mechanisms, such as specialized traps and toxic compounds, to infect and eliminate their nematode hosts [15, 16]. One notable example of a fungus that targets living nematodes is *Arthrobotrys oligospora* Fres., which shows significant promise as a biological control agent against parasitic plant nematodes [17, 18]. Its effectiveness stems from its antagonistic, parasitic, and predatory behaviors in the soil, relying on the complexity of the traps it forms to capture nematodes. *Arthrobotrys oligospora* can develop various mycelial structures for predation, including conidial traps, hyphal spirals, appressoria, and three-dimensional sticky networks [16, 19]. The initial step in capturing nematodes by *A. oligospora* involves the chemotaxis of fungal hyphae, which release volatile compounds to attract their prey [20, 21]. Additionally, the fungus produces antibiotics and toxic substances to digest the nematode' s organs and eliminate competing microorganisms. It also releases toxic terpene compounds that form the sticky substances used in traps [22]. The glue produced by nematophagous fungi is a sticky material composed of proteins and carbohydrates. These carbohydrates coat nematode surfaces and facilitate communication via chemotaxis and pectin. Specifically, *A. oligospora* recognizes nematodes through the pectin component Gal-Nac [23, 24]. Fungi compete for limited food resources and can often switch from a saprophytic lifestyle to a parasitic one. Laboratory experiments have demonstrated that a low carbon-to-nitrogen (C:N) ratio can trigger this transition from saprophytism to predation. Specifically, the addition of ammonia (NH3) within a specific concentration range, along with steroids such as lanosterol, ergosterol, phytosterol, β-sitosterol, or cortisone acetate, has been shown to stimulate trap formation in these fungi [23, 25, 26]. Conversely, high concentrations of carbon dioxide (51.0%), exposure to light, and phosphate levels above 30 μM have been found to inhibit trap formation. There may also be regional differences in the activity of various isolates of nematophagous fungi [27].

In Kyrgyzstan, little attention has been paid to studying these unique predatory fungi and their potential use against soil-dwelling parasitic nematodes, which cause significant crop production losses. Vegetable and field crops in many regions and climates are at risk from harmful stem and root nematodes. In recent years, large amounts of chemical nematicides, crop rotation practices, and resistant plant varieties have been employed to combat these parasitic nematodes. However, these methods have drawbacks, including environmental pollution, limited crop rotation options, and a shortage of resistant varieties. As a result, there is an urgent need for alternative control methods.

Isolating local predatory fungal strains with high activity to control parasitic nematodes in crops is essential as an alternative to chemical nematicides. Local species of predatory fungi are considered well-adapted to the climatic conditions of various regions' soil habitats.

The main aim of this study was to isolate predatory fungi from natural soil environments using classical and molecular biological methods and to select highly active strains against harmful parasitic nematodes.

2. Materials and methods

2.1 Isolation of nematodes for screening tests

To isolate the garlic nematode *Ditylenchus dipsaci*, the Baermann funnel technique was employed to extract it from garlic and potato samples. The isolated nematodes were maintained on cornmeal agar plates at 25°C. They were subcultured every 2 weeks and regularly monitored under a light microscope for morphological and viability characteristics. The garlic nematode, *Ditylenchus dipsaci,* was identified using the identification keys described in the sources by Mai and Mullin [28].

2.2 Isolation of predatory fungi from natural sources

A total of 50 samples, including crop residues, compost, and soil, were collected to isolate predatory fungi from various ecosystems in Kyrgyzstan (**Table 1**). The samples were gathered between September and November and April and June, spanning the years 2016 to 2019. Individual samples were placed in plastic bags and stored at 4°C until analysis. Modified versions of established methods were utilized to isolate *A. oligospora fungi* [29, 30]. Each sample was coarsely ground and thoroughly mixed using a blender.

To isolate the primary colonies of these fungi, a cornmeal agar medium (CMA) containing 1% streptomycin to inhibit bacterial growth was utilized. Three grams of a slurry composite sample were placed on the surface of the CMA. As bait, 100 healthy garlic nematodes (*Ditylenchus dipsaci*) were added to each plate, with a variation of ±32 (n = 3).

The plates were incubated at room temperature (26°C) for several weeks. The plates were examined under a dissecting microscope during the incubation, and fungal colonies were observed and recorded. Subsequently, fungal colonies were purified, and single-spore isolations were performed on CMA medium to obtain pure fungal cultures, and at least three subcultures were prepared. A specific microculture slide technique was employed to determine the shape and size of conidia, conidiophores, and other capturing structures. Taxa were identified morphologically using established identification keys [31, 32].

2.3 The solid and liquid media used to cultivate predatory fungi

Several nutrient media were used to determine the morphological and cultural properties of predatory fungi.

Habitats	Site #	Location	GPS coordinates
Potato field, plant residues	P-1, P-2, P-3, P-4, P-5	Jeti-Oguz district, Kyzyl-Suu village Issik-Kul region	42° 20′ 34.9188″ N 78° 0′ 18.9648″E
Potato grown soil	PS-1, PS-2,PS-3, PS-4, PS-5	Jeti-Oguz district Issik-Kul region	42° 20′ 34.9188″ N 78° 0′ 18.9648″ E
Potato field, potato tubers damaged by nematodes	PT-1, PT-2,PT-3, PT-4, PT-5, PT-6, PT-7, PT-8, PT-9, PT-10	Jeti-Oguz district Issik-Kul region	42° 19′ 49.98″ N 78° 14′ 23.04″ E
Compost is obtained by the decomposition of plant debris	C-1,C-2,C-3,C-4, C-5	Jany-Zher, Sokuluk district, Chui region	42.8573,74.2945
Debris	D-1, D-2,D-3, D-4, D-5	Jany-Zher, Sokuluk district, Chui region	42.8573,74.2945
Garlic grown soil	G-1, G-2, G-3, G-4, G-5	Jany-Zher, Sokuluk district, Chui region	42.8573,74.2945
Garlic grown soil	G-6, G-7, G-8, G-9, G-10	Experimental field of the Agriculture Faculty	42° 52′ 12.00″ N 74° 35′ 24.00″ E
Debris	D-6, D-7, D-8, D-9, D-10	Experimental field of the Agriculture Faculty	42° 52′ 12.00″ N 74° 35′ 24.00″ E

Table 1.
Examples of locations and natural materials for isolating predatory fungi [29].

Corn agar: Corn flour 20.0 g; agar-agar 15 g; distilled water 1 L; pH 6.2; *Czapek medium:* Sucrose 20.0 g; NaNO3 2 g; KH2PO4 1 g; MgSO4 × 7H2O 0.5 g; KCl 0.5 g; FeSO4 0.01 g; agar-agar 20 g; distilled water 1 L; pH 6.5;

Rice and sorghum medium: Rice 15 g; sorghum 15 g; distilled water 200 mL; pH 7.2.

Richard's medium: Sucrose 50 g; KNO3 10 g; K2HPO4 5 g; MgSO4 × 7H2O 0.5 g; FeCl3 0.02 g; pH 6.0;

Yeast extract, peptone, and soluble starch medium: Soluble starch 20 g; yeast extract 4 g; K2HPO4 0.5 g; MgSO4 × 7H2O 0.2 g; pH 7.0.

2.4 In vitro test for evaluation of fungal activity against living nematodes

A piece (5 mm in diameter) was cut from the margin of *A. oligospora* fungal colonies and transferred to the centre of a Petri dish containing 1.5% water agar medium. The Petri dishes were incubated in the dark at 25°C for 1 week.

Following this incubation, the Petri dishes were inoculated with a 1 ml suspension of *Ditylenchus dipsaci* nematodes containing 100 to 150 individuals. Four to five drops of the nematode suspension were distributed around the fungal colonies.

Control plates that did not contain fungi or nematodes were also prepared. The formation of traps was observed and recorded under a stereomicroscope (EMZ-5 with Swf10x, MEIJI, Zoom Stereo Microscope, Japan). The average number of trap rings formed was calculated for 10 randomly selected microscopic fields. Four replicates were conducted to evaluate trap formation over 96 hours. Microscopic images were captured using an ML5000 MEIJI TECHNO microscope fitted with a Euromex CMEX-32000 digital camera system.

2.5 Evaluation of fungal activity on live nematodes in the rhizosphere soil of potato plants

For the assessment of fungal activity against nematodes, three pots per treatment containing mixed soil and humus in a 3:1 ratio were utilized.

Potato buds were planted at a depth of 5 to 6 cm in pots. The colonies of *A. oligospora*, in the form of 5 mm diameter disks, were mixed with soil—four fungal colony disks per 500 g of soil—and incubated at 25°C in the dark for 1 week under sterile conditions.

Three experimental options were introduced to assess the effectiveness of predatory fungi against nematodes in the potato root system:

Control 1: Plants without any treatment, nematodes, or nematophagous fungi. Control 2: Plants with introduced nematodes but without nematophagous fungi. In these control pots, 1 ml of a suspension containing mixed life stages of the nematode *Ditylenchus dipsaci* (approximately 1000 worms) was added to the soil, which was then incubated under natural conditions.

Experiment 3: In this option, 1 ml of a suspension containing mixed life stages of *Ditylenchus dipsaci* (1000 worms) was added to each pot, along with the planted material. When the potato leaves developed, the predatory fungi were introduced into the soil. For this, 5 mm-diameter discs of *A. oligospora* colonies (four pieces) were mixed with the soil and incubated in sterile, dark conditions at room temperature for 1 week. We believe that, during this period and under these conditions, the interaction between nematophagous fungi and nematodes would be intensified in the soil surrounding the potato root system.

In the fourth experiment, a 1 ml suspension containing mixed life stages of the nematode *Ditylenchus dipsaci* (totaling 1000 worms) was added to the soil. Unlike the plots in the third experiment, in this case, nematophagous fungi were introduced into the soil around the potato root at the time the seed material was planted and again as the leaves began to develop.

2.6 DNA extraction, marker sequence determination and phylogenetic reconstruction

For DNA extraction, fungal isolates were cultivated on Potato Dextrose Agar (PDA) and Yeast Extract Agar at 25°C. Approximately 100 mg of mycelium was placed into a screw-capped 2 ml microcentrifuge tube containing Lysing Matrix C (MP Biomedicals). DNA was extracted using the DNeasy Plant Kit (Qiagen).

Purified DNA was eluted in 100 μL of elution buffer AE and stored at −20° C. DNA sequences were amplified from fungal DNA samples using standard Taq DNA polymerase (New England Biolabs) and the PCR primers listed in **Table 2**. This process targeted internal partial sequences of several genes: the EF-1α gene, which encodes the translation elongation factor 1-alpha; the RPB2 gene, which encodes the second-largest subunit of RNA polymerase II; and the TUBB gene, which encodes beta-tubulin. Additionally, the complete ribosomal RNA (rrn) operon internal transcribed spacer (ITS) region was amplified, encompassing the ITS1 and ITS2 elements along with the 5.8S rRNA encoding sequence.

To clarify the molecular taxonomy of the KTMU-7 isolate, we compared it with known Arthrobotrys reference sequences from Yang et al. [33]. The sequences

Primer designation	Primer sequence	Annealing temperature (°C)	Elongation time (sec)
ITS4	5′-TCCTCCGCTTATTGATATGC	52	60
ITS5	5′-GGAAGTAAAAGTCGTAACAAGG		
EF1A-983F	5′-GCYCCYGGHCAYCGTGAYTTYAT	52	120
EF1A-2218R	5′-ATGACACCRACRGCRACRGTYTG		
EF1A-1567R	5′-ACHGTRCCRATACCACCSATCTT	Sequencing primer	
RPB2-5f	5′-GAYGAYMGWGATCAYTTYGG	58	120
RPB2-7r	5′-CCCATRGCTTGYTTRCCCAT		
RPB2-6f	5′-TGGGGKWTGGTYTGYCCTGC	Sequencing primer	
Bt2a	5′-CTGCCCAGTGCTCTGAATGTC	52	60
Bt2b	5′-GCTGAATTACCATTGCGGAGAGG		

Table 2.
Oligonucleotide primers and reaction-specific PCR parameters used in this study [29].

generated for the KTMU-7 isolate were used to search GenBank for highly homologous entries. The advanced software tool BLASTn [34] facilitated the search. Among the top 100 hits, sorted by descending maximum identity value, those with at least 80% sequence coverage that were assigned to the genus Arthrobotrys were included in the reference dataset.

2.7 Data analysis

The occurrence frequency (F) of *A. oligospora* and the total number of fungal isolates from each natural habitat were calculated using the following formula, based on the total number of all species.

$$F = \frac{\text{Individual number of species}}{\text{Individual number of all species}} \times 100 \tag{1}$$

If an individual species was isolated from any of the three replicates, it was deemed to have one occurrence. All statistical analyses were carried out using the Statistical Package for the Social Sciences (SPSS). Statistical significance was defined at an alpha level of 0.05.

3. Results

3.1 Sampling sites

The locations where samples were collected are detailed in **Table 1**.

3.2 Isolation of garlic endoparasitic nematodes

Identification of nematodes obtained from diseased roots and stems of garlic and potato was conducted using the Determination book [35, 36], and they were morphologically confirmed as *Ditylenchus dipsaci*. Morphological characteristics of this species include the following: the female body length ranges from 1 to 1.8 mm, while the male body length varies from 1.2 to 1.5 mm. The stylet length is between 10 and 12 μm (**Figure 1**). The female lays approximately 200–300 eggs. An egg measures 67 to 88 μm in length and 25 to 34 μm in width; the second-stage larvae measure 0.3 mm, and the fourth-stage larvae range from 0.96 to 1.28 mm. The nematode population obtained was maintained at room temperature for further experimental use.

Garlic nematodes are widespread in all garlic-growing regions of Kyrgyzstan, particularly in the Issyk-Kul and Chui areas. These nematodes invade leaves and stalks, acting as parasites and damaging roots. At +15°C, the generation time is 19–23 days.

3.3 Isolation of predatory fungi

To ensure long-term viability, the primary colonies of predatory fungi were cultivated using three methods under laboratory conditions: (1) the samples were plated on a solid medium measuring 10 x 10 mm; (2) the samples were combined with live nematodes and placed on solid medium; and (3) the samples were suspended in water containing nematodes. Although all three methods resulted in colony growth, the most effective technique involved mixing the samples with nematodes on solid medium and suspending them in water with nematodes.

From various natural sources studied, approximately 40 primary colonies were obtained. Within a week, these suspected colonies were transferred to a pure medium to facilitate subculturing and obtain a pure culture of the sought fungus. Ultimately, twelve strains of predatory fungi were isolated.

The prevalence of *A. oligospora* in natural substrates varied significantly. The highest incidence of this fungus was recorded in the residues of damaged potatoes collected from the Jeti-Oguz district, specifically in Kyzyl-Suu village in the Issyk-Kul region, at 36.0 ± 0.091% ($P \leq 0.05$). Additionally, garlic crops exhibited a notable population of *A. oligospora*; in the Sokuluk district of the Chui region, the occurrence

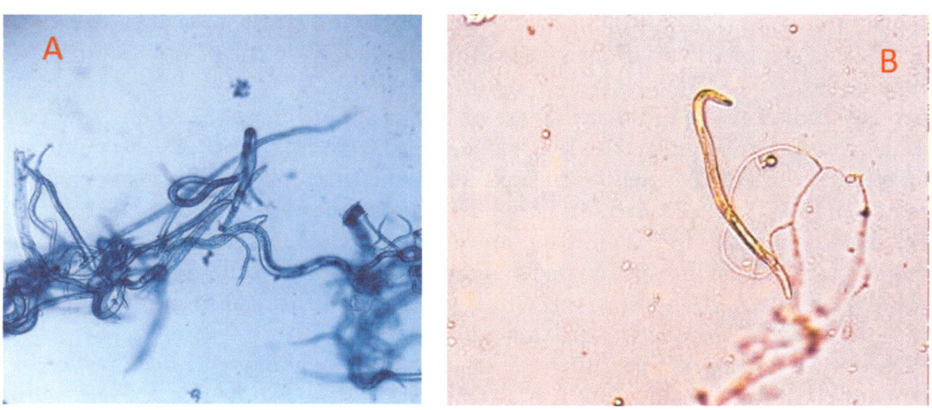

Figure 1.
Ditylenchus dipsaci *isolated from infested potatoes (A) and infected garlic (B).*

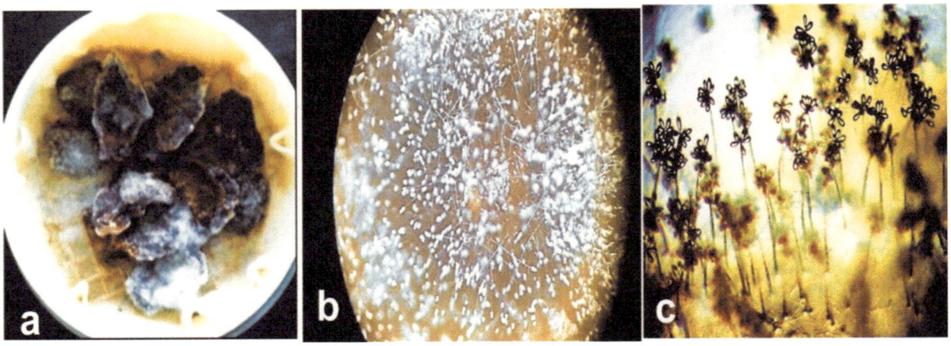

Figure 2.
Primary colonies of Arthrobotrys oligospora *from damaged potatoes and the emergence of conidiophores. a:– the onset of growth of white, fluffy mycelium covering potato tubers; b, c: emergence of conidiophores growing upwards upon visual observation [29].*

was observed at 20.0 ± 0.87%. The garlic-grown soils of the experimental station of the Agriculture Faculty exhibited a fungal frequency of 14.0 ± 0.67% ($P \leq 0.05$). In the decomposed plant debris, the frequency of fungi was low, at −10.0 ± 0.51% ($P \leq 0.05$). The frequency of *A. oligospora* was particularly low in wild plant residues, reaching only 6.0 ± 0.37% ($P \leq 0.05$).

Figure 2 depicts the isolated primary colonies of *A. oligospora* from damaged potatoes, along with the conidio-forming mycelium of the fungus.

3.4 Morphological characteristics of *A. oligospora* isolates

As demonstrated by microscopy (×40, ×100), the obtained isolates exhibit branched vegetative hyphae and a mycelial structure. Conidiophores grow vertically, are pretty long, and their lengths reach 27,270 ± 0.02 μm (n = 50). At the blunt ends of the conidiophores, at the tips of the sterigmata, two-celled, pear- shaped, transparent conidia develop. The average size of the conidia was 27.2 x 16.1 ± 0.031 μm (n = 50) (**Figure 3**). A single conidiophore branch can produce more than six conidia, which form successive clusters.

Some studies have noted that spores of predatory fungi increase in size when exposed to nematodes [37], whereas others have observed a decrease in spore size under similar conditions [38]. In our research, we found that spores of *Arthrobotrys* spp. cultures exhibited variations in size and morphology in the presence and absence of nematodes.

In our studies, we found that the size of fungal spores increases when grown on CMA medium; for instance, they reach (31–51 ± 0.019 μm, n = 50). When cultured on a mixed medium (CMA + peptone), both distal and proximal conidia also exhibit larger sizes (30–51 ± 0.23 μm). As noted by other studies [39, 40], fungal conidia attached to nematodes in the wild are larger and more elongated (31–51 ± 0.17 μm). These data are consistent with ours. To obtain larger spores of these fungi, we selected a mixed medium (CMA + peptone), which yields greater fungal spore biomass and may be more effective against nematodes.

It is known that predatory fungi can form chlamydospores with thick cell walls under unfavorable environmental conditions. Other studies note that these structures play a crucial role in the predatory lifestyle of these fungi. Unlike saprophytic fungi, these predatory fungi require additional stimulation to produce chlamydospores. In

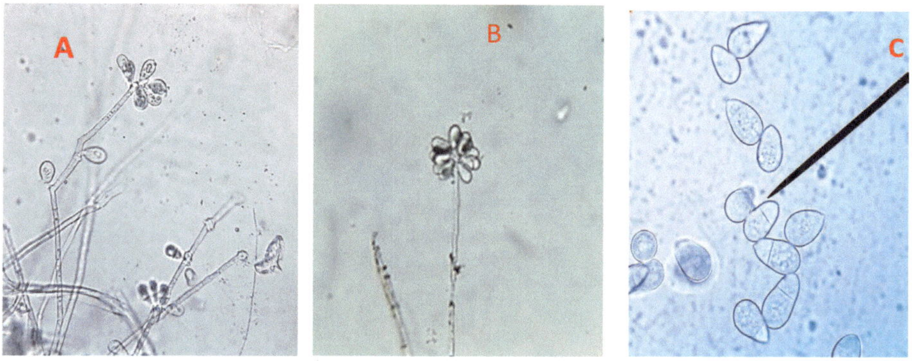

Figure 3.
Morphology of Arthrobotrys oligospora *(isolate KTMU-7) observed under light microscopy, ×40. (A, B) Conidia are located at the apex of conidiophores; (C) two-celled, pear-shaped conidia. Adapted from Ref. [29].*

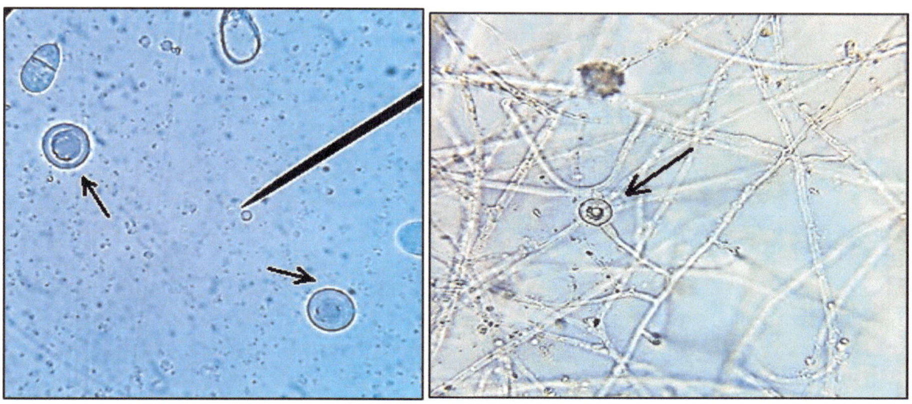

Figure 4.
Chlamydospores produced by Arthrobotrys oligospora *(isolate KTMU-7) in CMA after 15 days of incubation [29].*

our studies, we generated intercalary, ellipsoidal chlamydospores on plates containing 2% CMA after 15–18 days of incubation (**Figure 4**).

3.5 Screening of fungi for predatory activity against live nematodes in vitro

For the application of such fungi in biological control in the field, nematophagous activity must first be screened in vitro. Microscopic observation of slides of co-incubated fungi and nematodes revealed the emergence of a single trapping ring in the fungi, which, over time, were able to form fully developed three-dimensional trapping structures and networks. *A. oligospora* began to trap nematodes 24 hours after the inoculation of fungal cultures. The number of traps and the percentage of nematodes captured by the fungus increased over time (**Figure 5**).

Microscopic observation revealed that, within the first 24 hours, trapping rings and nets began to form on the fungal mycelium originating from the conidia. By 48–72 hours, trap formation intensified, and their numbers increased. Consequently, the number of nematodes captured by the predatory fungi also rose. Nematodes already sedentary in the trap became immobile within 6–10 hours (**Figure 6a-d**). By 96 hours,

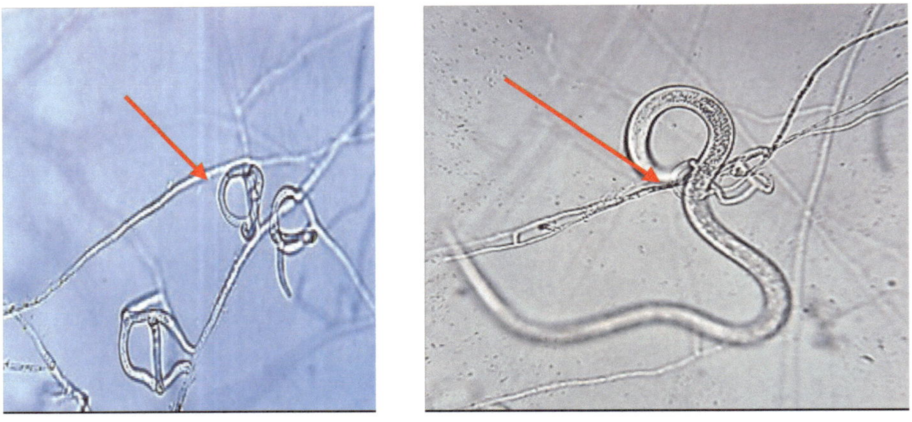

Figure 5.
Adhesive network trap formed by A. oligospora *fungi: single ring trap (A) at 24 h and traps containing captured nematodes at 30 h (B).*

active penetration and germination of the fungal mycelium within the body cavity of the nematodes became noticeable. Even after the nematodes were released from the traps, parts of the mycelium still attached to their surfaces could grow and release mycelium into the environment. By 122 hours, the fungal mycelium had multiplied inside the nematodes, completely dissolving their internal contents and leaving behind only traces (**Figure 6f**).

Microscopic observation revealed that within the first 24 hours, trapping rings and nets began to form on the fungal mycelium g rowing from the conidia. By 48–72 hours, trap formation had intensified and their number had increased, and, accordingly, the number of nematodes caught by the predatory fungi also increased. Nematodes already sedentary in the trap became immobile within 6–10 hours (**Figure 6a-d**). By 96 hours, active penetration and germination of the fungal mycelium inside the body cavity of the nematodes was noticeable. Microscopic observation revealed that within the first 24 hours, trapping rings and nets began to form on the fungal mycelium growing from the conidia. By 48–72 hours, trap formation had intensified and their number had increased, and, accordingly, the number of nematodes caught by the predatory fungi also increased. Nematodes already sedentary in the trap became immobile within 6–10 h ours (**Figure 6a-d**). By 96 hours, active penetration and germination of the fungal mycelium inside the body cavity of the nematodes was noticeable. Even when the nematodes were released from the traps, part of the mycelium that remained attached to their surface was able to grow and release mycelium into the environment. By 122 hours, the fungal mycelium had multiplied inside the nematodes, completely dissolving their internal contents and leaving behind only traces (**Figure 6f**). Even when the nematodes were released from the traps, part of the mycelium that remained attached to their surface was able to grow and release mycelium into the environment. By 122 hours, the fungal mycelium had multiplied inside the nematodes, completely dissolving their internal contents and leaving behind only traces (**Figure 6f**).

Joint cultivation of in vitro fungi *A. oligospora* and *D. dipsaci* was conducted using 1.5% water agar to investigate the formation of trapping rings in predatory fungi in the presence of nematodes; in the control group, tap water was used instead of a

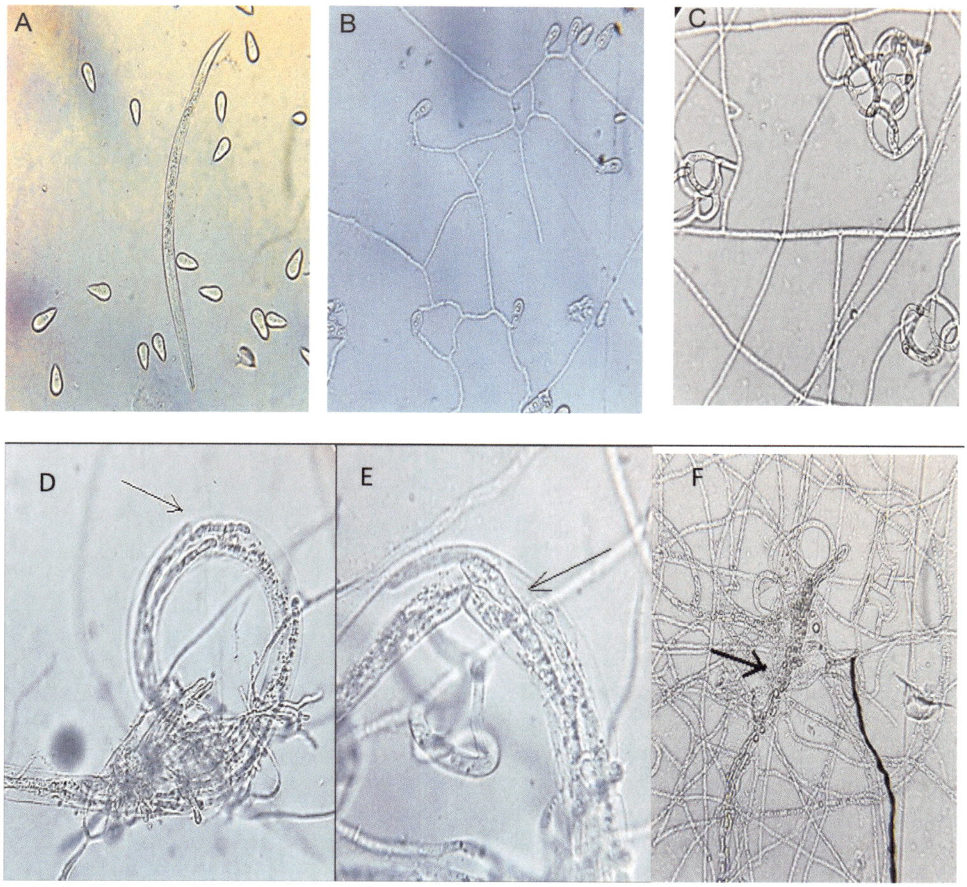

Figure 6.
Nematode along the fungi conidia (A); trapping rings and nets began to form on the fungal mycelium growing from conidia (B, C); growth of mycelium of the fungus Arthrobotrys oligospora *inside a nematode larva (D, E); digestion of nematode larvae by the fungus* Arthrobotrys oligospora *(F). Adapted from Ref. [29].*

nematode suspension. The average number of traps formed in contact with nematodes was counted across 10 fields of view under the microscope. These calculations, performed in ten replicates, showed that the number of traps formed positively correlated with the duration of the previous joint incubation, with values of 39.25 ± 2.14 after 24 h, 157.50 ± 2.9 after 48 h, and 257.50 ± 4.17 after 96 h ($P < 0.05$). In the control experiments, traps were also formed, but their number was 5–10 times lower than in the experimental group, specifically, 12.25 ± 1.20 after 24 h, 17.50 ± 3.97 after 48 h, and 28.75 ± 9.07 after 96 h ($P < 0.05$) (**Figure 7**). Therefore, these results demonstrate that live nematodes enhance the active and dense formation of traps in predatory fungi.

3.6 Determination of the predatory activity of *A. oligospora* fungi in soil conditions: in the rhizosphere of potato plants

The results of the combined incubation of *A. oligospora* fungi and the parasitic nematodes *D. dipsaci* in the rhizosphere soil of potato plants showed significant

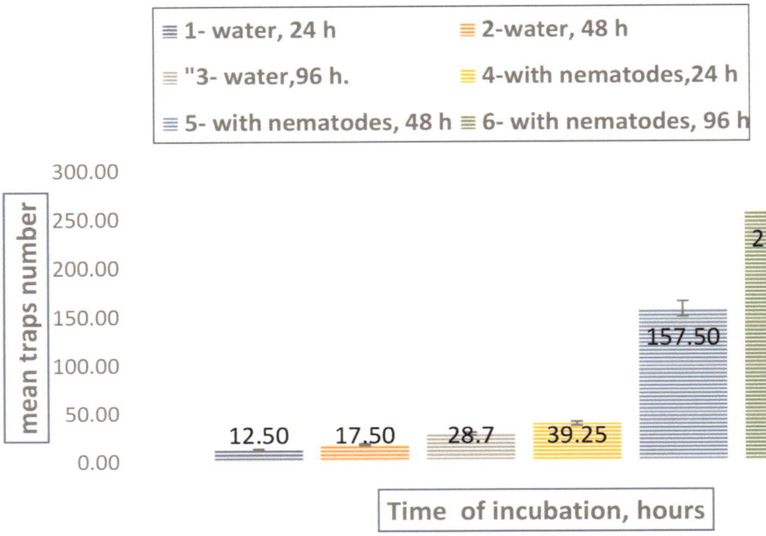

Figure 7.
Means of traps for A. oligospora *induced by* Ditylenchus dipsaci *garlic nematodes for 96 h (n = 10; P < 0.05). EMBED Excel.Chart.8.*

differences between the variants and the control groups. In the control group, which was not exposed to either nematodes or predatory fungi, the above-ground and below-ground organs of the potato displayed no pathological symptoms: the stems were straight and thick, and the leaf blades were a rich green, free of any spots (**Figure 8a**). In contrast, plants exposed to nematodes without any suspensions of predatory fungi for protection exhibited clear pathological symptoms: the stems became weak and thin, and the leaf blades were small and yellowing (**Figure 8b**). Conversely, when plants were exposed to nematodes along with a single treatment of carnivorous fungi, the stems were of medium thickness, the leaves showed no visible signs of disease, and the plants maintained a normal height (**Figure 8c**). Following the second treatment, the agronomic parameters of the plants improved further: no disease symptoms were observed, the leaves and stems were of medium thickness and standard size, and the plants developed better than in the other experiments (**Figure 8d**).

Upon examination of the underground organs, root hair nematode infestation was evident. In contrast, the roots of control plants that were not exposed to nematodes were thick, exhibited no symptoms of disease, and had begun to form tubers. However, the roots of nematode-exposed plants without fungal treatment failed to form tubers and instead disintegrated into thin strands. Additionally, the lateral roots of potato plants exposed to nematodes in combination with one or two treatments of *A. oligospora* formed tubers and displayed no symptoms of disease; after two applications of the carnivorous fungus, the roots of these plants appeared healthier overall and were thicker than those of plants treated only once.

3.7 Field testing of predatory fungi against nematodes

For this experiment, we used three strains known to be effective in the laboratory. Following the scheme outlined below, we applied 1 and 2% liquid preparations of

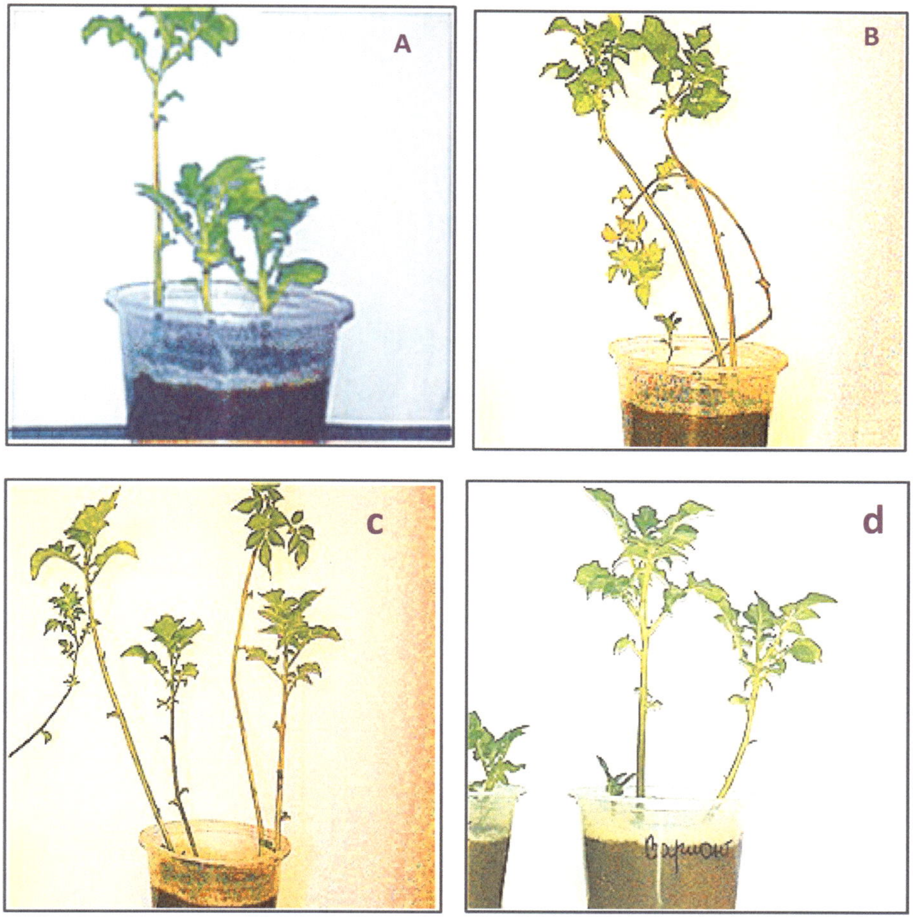

Figure 8.
Potato plants from in vivo experiments evaluating the biocontrol capacity of A. oligospora *KTMU-7 include untreated control plants (A); plants exposed to* D. dipsaci *nematodes but not treated with fungi (B); plants exposed to* D. dipsaci *nematodes and treated once with* A. oligospora *(C); and plants exposed to* D. dipsaci *nematodes and treated twice with* A. oligospora *(D) [29].*

fungi to the nematode-infected garlic field. As illustrated in **Figure 9**, we introduced the predatory fungi to the garlic field at the beginning, middle, and end of the experimental area. We compared the results with those from the control group.

When introducing a 1–2% suspension of the predatory fungus into the garlic field at the start of treatment, 36–37 ± 0.01 garlic nematodes per soil sample were counted in the initial part of the experimental area. After treatment, 7–8 ± 0.01 nematodes were found 7 days later. In the middle of the field before treatment, there were 45–46 ± 0.01 nematodes, and after treatment, their numbers dropped to between 5 and 10 ± 0.01. At the end of the field, 50–51 ± 0.01 nematodes were counted before treatment, which decreased to 5–10 ± 0.01 afterwards. In contrast, the control variant showed an increase in nematode numbers from 34 to 58 ± 0.01 within 7 days (**Table 3**). These data demonstrate the effectiveness of three strains of *Arthrobotrys oligospora* under field conditions against garlic nematodes. Considering various negative abiotic factors in the environment, a 2% suspension of predatory fungi can be

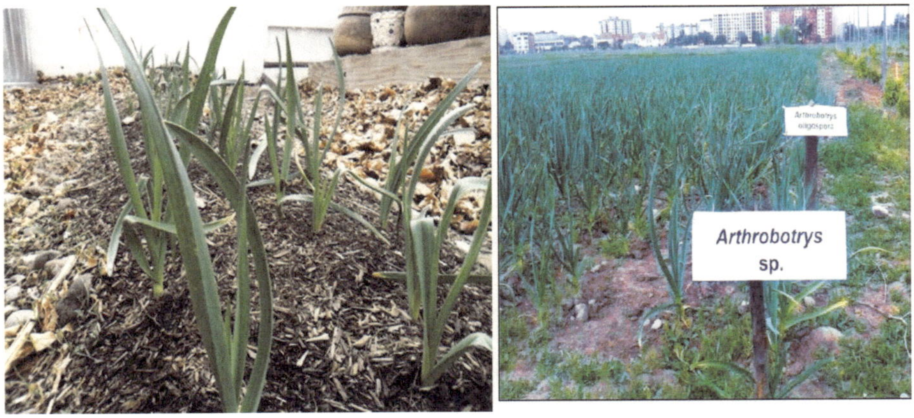

Figure 9.
Field testing of predatory fungi activity.

#	Predatory fungi	Applied dose of fungi	Nematodes per gram of soil before treatment			Nematodes per gram of soil following treatment		
			The beginning of the field	The middle part	The end of the field	The beginning of the field	The middle part	The end of the field
1	*Arthrobotrys oligospora*	1.0% of suspension	34	34	40	5 ± 0.01	8 ± 0.01	8 ± 0.01
2	*Arthrobotrys* spp	1.0% of suspension	34	35	39	4 ± 0.01	5 ± 0.01	6 ± 0.01
3	Control	Water	34	35	37	39 ± 0.01	39 ± 0.01	40 ± 0.01
4	*Arthrobotrys oligospora*	2.0% of suspension	34	34	40	1 ± 0.01	2 ± 0.01	4 ± 0.01
	Arthrobotrys spp.	2.0% of suspension	34	34	40	1 ± 0.01	2 ± 0.01	4 ± 0.01

Table 3.
Activity of predatory fungi against nematodes in the soil surrounding garlic roots (n = 3).

recommended; the higher the density of their traps in the soil, the more favorable the results of biological control will be.

Some studies have indicated that environmental conditions may influence nematophagous fungi. Taking this into account, we recommend that a 2% preparation is suitable for pre-treating garlic under field conditions or for spraying during the growing season.

3.8 Molecular taxonomic characterization of the nematophagous fungal isolate KTMU-7

Consensus marker sequences of 602 bp (ITS), 213 bp (ef1a), 275 bp (tubB), and 705 bp (rpb2) were obtained by assembling raw sequence data from genomic DNA isolated from a pure culture of fungal isolate KTMU-7. These sequences have been

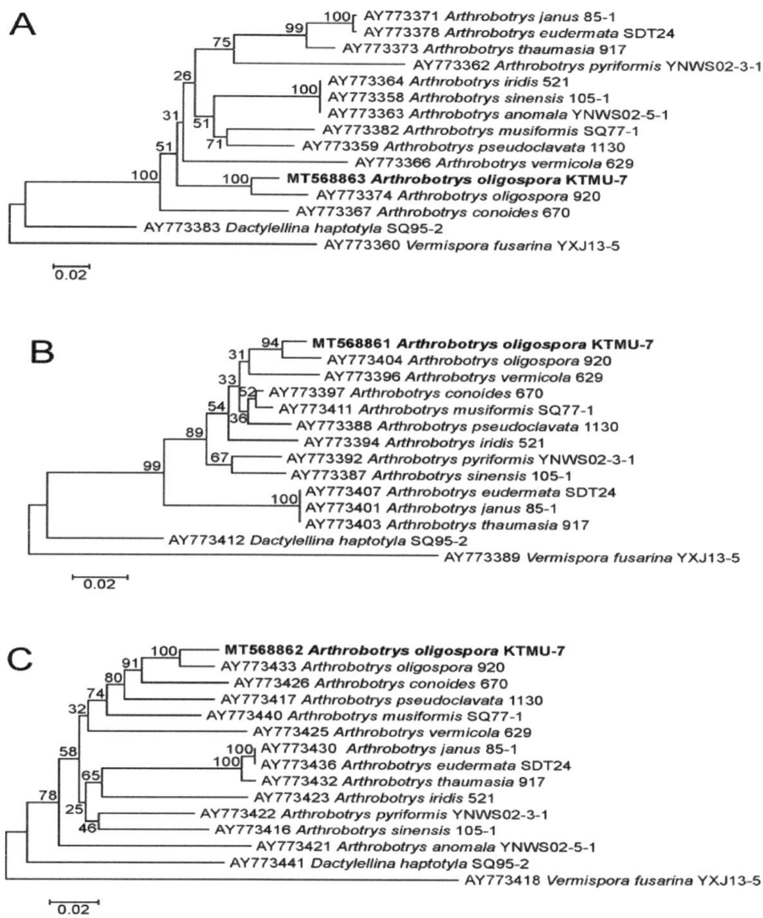

Figure 10.
Neighbor-joining (NJ) phylogeny of Arthrobotrys *fungi reconstructed from β-tubulin (tubB) (A), translation elongation factor 1α (ef1a) (B), and RNA polymerase II (rpb2) and (C) encoding sequences. The GenBank accession number, genus, species, and strain designations label terminal branches. The isolate under study is shown in bold. Numbers on internal branches indicate bootstrap support percentages. Size bars correspond to 2% sequence divergence along horizontal branches. Orthologous sequences from the closely related nematophagous fungal genus* Dactylellina *have been used as an internal standard delimiting genus boundaries, while orthologs from the more distantly related fungus Vermispora are included and serve as outgroup to root the tree [29].*

submitted to Genbank under accession numbers MT559369 and MT568861–MT568863. When queried against the Barcode of Life database, the ITS consensus displayed the highest similarity (96.9–100%) to members of the fungal species *Arthrobotrys oligospora*. All four consensus sequences identified as top matches in the Genbank records were assigned to the genus Arthrobotrys when used as a query in a BlastN search. In four single-marker phylogenies reconstructed from aligned nucleotide sequences (**Figure 10**), the sequence from isolate KTMU-7 was most closely related to orthologs representing the taxonomic species *Arthrobotrys oligospora*, with the corresponding clade receiving relatively high bootstrap support values of 100% (rpb2, tubB), 99% (ITS), and 94% (ef1a). For the ITS marker, pairwise sequence similarity between the KTMU-7 sequence and reference sequences, determined using a p-distance matrix (data not shown), ranged from identical to 96.7% within the putative *A. oligospora* clade. In contrast, the most closely related reference sequences outside this clade did not demonstrate similarity greater than 94.5%. These genetic data support the classification of KTMU-7 as a taxonomic species of the fungus *Arthrobotrys oligospora*.

4. Conclusions

An analysis of the literature on the fauna and harmful effects of phytonematodes across various agricultural regions revealed that these soil parasites cause significant damage to crops. To develop non-chemical methods for protecting agricultural crops from parasitic nematodes, this study explored alternative approaches. One promising alternative to chemical nematicides is a predatory fungus, which has demonstrated effectiveness against phytonematodes, including *D. dipsaci*, in both experimental and field trials. The isolate KTMU-7, identified as *Arthrobotrys oligospora*, was first isolated and described morphologically and molecularly in Kyrgyzstan. This strain (KTMU-7) effectively eradicated up to 85.7% of garlic nematodes from the rhizosphere soil of potted potato plants and field garlic crops. This positions it as a potentially valuable resource for developing biological control agents against nematodes.

Author details

Tinatin Doolotkeldieva
Kyrgyz National Agrarian University named after K.I. Skryabin, Plant Protection Centre, Bishkek City, Kyrgyzstan

*Address all correspondence to: tdoolotkeldieva@gmail.com

References

[1] Dzhunusov KK. Phytohelminths of agrocenoses of Kyrgyzstan. Manas Journal of Agriculture and Life Sciences (MJAL). 2015;**5**(1):13-19 (In Russian)

[2] Azamat Kyzy K, Shekekov AS. Soil entomopathogenic nematodes of the biogeocenosis of the Chui Valley. Journal of Science, New Technologies and Innovations of Kyrgyzstan. 2021;**2**:2419 (In Russian)

[3] Chakaeva AS. Sugar beet nematode in Kyrgyzstan and substantiation of methods of control. In: Dissertation and Abstract According to the Higher Attestation Commission of the Russian Federation 03.00.20. Moscow; 1984 (In Russian)

[4] Dzhunusov KK. Influence of Phytonematodes on Productivity of Crops. Bishkek: News of Universities; 2014. p. 12 (In Russian)

[5] Dzhunusov KK, Sodombekov IS. Ecological and taxonomic analysis of the Kyrgyzstan's nematode fauna of vegetable crops. Advances in Modern Natural Science. 2016;**1**:71-77 (In Russian)

[6] Dzhunusov KK. Phytohelminths of agrocenoses of Kyrgyzstan. News of Universities of Kyrgyzstan. 2015;**10**:5 (In Russian)

[7] Nurbekkyzy M, Shekekov A. The role of crop rotation in reducing the number of parasitic nematodes in Alfalfa's root soil and root system. Science, New Technologies and Innovations of Kyrgyzstan. 2023. DOI: 10.26104/NNTIK (In Russian)

[8] Janssen GJW. The relevance of races in *Ditylenchus dipsaci* (Kühn) Filipjev, the stem nematode. Fundamental and Applied Nematology. 1994;**5**:469-473

[9] Aftalion B, Cohn E. Characterization of two races of the stem and bulb nematode (*Ditylenchus dipsaci*) in Israel. Phytoparasitica. 1990;**18**:229-232

[10] Song W, Dai M, Shi Q, Liang C, Duan F, Zhao H. Diagnosis and characterization of Ditylenchus destructor isolated from *Mazus japonicus* in China. Life (Basel). 2023;**13**(8):1758. DOI: 10.3390/life13081758

[11] Chitwood DJ. Research on plant-parasitic nematode biology conducted by the United States Department of Agriculture-Agricultural Research Service. Pest Management Science. 2003;**59**(6–7):748-753. DOI: 10.1002/ps.684

[12] Capizzi-Banas S, Deloge M, Remy M, Schwartzbrod J. Liming as an advanced treatment for sludge sanitisation: Helminth eggs elimination—Ascaris eggs as model. Water Research. 2004;**38**:3251-3258

[13] Palomero AM, Cazapal-Monteiro CF, Valderrábano E, Paz-Silva A, Sánchez- Andrade R, Arias MS. Soil fungi enable the control of gastrointestinal nematodes in wild bovidae captive in a zoological park: A 4-year trial. Parasitology. 2020;**147**:791-798

[14] Saumell CA, Fernández AS, Fusé LA, Rodríguez M, Sagüés MF, Iglesias LE. Nematophagous fungi from decomposing cattle faeces in Argentina. Revista Iberoamericana de Micología. 2015;**32**:252-256. DOI: 10.1016/j.riam

[15] Karaka SM. Nematode-destroying fungi: Infection structures, interaction mechanisms and biocontrol. Communications Faculty of Sciences University of Ankara Series C Biology. 2020;**29**:176-201. Available from: https://

dergipark.org.tr/en/pub/communc/issue/51836/672275

[16] Wang D, Ma N, Rao W, Zhang Y. Recent advances in life history transition with nematode-trapping fungus *Arthrobotrys oligospora* and its application in sustainable agriculture. Pathogens. 2023;**12**:367. DOI: 10.3390/pathogens12030367

[17] Dong LQ, Zhang KQ. Microbial control of plant-parasitic nematodes: A five-party interaction. Plant and Soil. 2006;**288**:31-45

[18] Van OC. Fungal pathogenesis: Hungry fungus eats nematode. Nature Reviews Microbiology. 2011;**9**:766-767

[19] Swe A, Jeewon R, Pointing SB, Hyde KD. Diversity and abundance of nematode trapping fungi from decaying litter in terrestrial, freshwater and mangrove habitats. Biodiversity and Conservation. 2009;**18**:1695-1714. DOI: 10.1007/s10531-008-9553-7

[20] Bargmann CI, Horvitz HR. Chemosensory neurons with overlapping functions direct chemotaxis to multiple chemicals in *C. elegans*. Neuron. 1991;**7**:729-742. DOI: 10.1016/0896-6273(91)90276-6

[21] Bargmann CI. Chemosensation in *C. elegans*. New York, NY, USA: WormBook; 2006. p. 129. DOI: 10.1895/wormbook.1.123.1

[22] Hsueh YP, Mahanti P, Schroeder FC, Sternberg PW. Nematode-trapping fungi eavesdrop on nematode pheromones. Current Biology. 2013;**23**:83-86. DOI: 10.1016/j.cub.2012.11.035

[23] Nguyen VL, Bastow JL, Jaffee BA, Strong DR. Response of nematode-trapping fungi to organic substrates in a coastal grassland soil. Mycological Research. 2007;**111**:856-862. DOI: 10.1016/j.mycres.2007.04.009

[24] Hsueh YP, Gronquist MR, Schwarz EM, Nath RD, Lee CH, Gharib S, et al. Nematophagous fungus *Arthrobotrys oligospora* mimics olfactory cues of sex and food to lure its nematode prey. Genomics and Evolutionary Biology Neuroscience. Elife. 18 Jan 2017; **6**:e20023. DOI: 10.7554/eLife.20023

[25] Lee JK, Kim DG, Lee SB. Nutritional requirements and mass production of nematode-trapping fungus, *Arthrobotrys oligospora*. Journal of Asia-Pacific Entomology. 2004;**7**:325-329. DOI: 10.1016/S1226-8615(08)60234-4

[26] Jaffee BA, Strong DR. Strong bottom-up and weak top-down effect in soil: Nematode-parasitized insects and nematode-trapping fungi. Soil Biology and Biochemistry. 2005;**37**:1011-1021. DOI: 10.1016/j.soilbio.2004.05.026

[27] Araújo JV, Mota MA, Campos AK. Controle biológico de helmintos parasitos de animais por fungos nematófagos. Revista Brasileira de Parasitologia Veterinária. 2004;**13**:165-170

[28] Mai WF, Mullin PG. Plant parasitic nematode. In: A Pictorial Key to Genera. 5th ed. Ithaca, New York: Cornell University Press; 1996. ISBN.1501728415, 9781501728419

[29] Doolotkeldieva T, Bobushova S, Muratbekova A, et al. Isolation, identification, and characterization of the nematophagous fungus *Arthrobotrys oligospora* from Kyrgyzstan. Acta Parasitologica. 2021;**66**:1349-1365. DOI: 10.1007/s11686-021-00404-5

[30] Wang FH, Xu Q, Wang BB, Wang KY, Xue YJ, Cai B, et al. Isolation,

identification and characterisation of the nematophagous fungus *Arthrobotrys thaumasia* (*Monacrosporium thaumasium*) from China. Biocontrol Science and Technology. 2017;**27**(3): 378-392. DOI: 10.1080/09583157.2017.1291908

[31] Li TF, Zhang KQ, Liu XZ. Taxonomy of Nematophagous Fungi. Beijing: Chinese Science and Technical Publishing; 2000

[32] Liu YJ, Whelen S, Hall BD. Phylogenetic relationships among ascomycetes: Evidence from an RNA polymerase II subunit. Molecular Biology and Evolution. 1999;**16**(12):1799-1808

[33] Yang Y, Yang E, An Z, Liu X. Evolution of nematode-trapping cells of predatory fungi of the Orbiliaceae based on evidence from rRNA-encoding DNA and multiprotein sequences. PNAS. 2007;**104**:8379-8384. DOI: 10.1073/pnas.0702770104

[34] Zhang Z, Schwartz S, Wagner L, Miller W. A greedy algorithm for aligning DNA sequences. Journal of Computational Biology. 2000;7:203-214

[35] Maggenti AR. General nematode morphology. In: Nickel WR, editor. Manual of Agricultural Nematology. New York: Marcel Dekker; 1991. pp. 1-46. ISBN-13: 978-0-8247-8397-6 (hbk) ISBN-13: 978-0-367-40297-6 (pbk)

[36] Kepenekci İ. Nematology (Plant Parasite and Entomopathogenic Nematodes) [General Nematology (Volume-I), Taxonomic Nematology (Volume-II)]. Ankara: Agricultural Science Series Publication; 2012

[37] Drechsler C. Some hyphomycetes that prey on free-living terricolous nematodes. Mycologia. 1937;**29**(4): 447-552. DOI: 10.1080/00275514.1937.12017222

[38] Haard K. Taxonomic studies on the genus *Arthrobotrys corda*. Mycologia. 1968;**60**(6):1140-1159. DOI: 10.2307/3757214

[39] Ojeda-Robertos NF, Torres-Acosta JFJ, Ayala-Burgos AJ, Sandoval-Castro CA, Valero Coss RO, Mendoza-de-Gives P. Digestibility of *Duddingtonia flagrans* chlamydospores in rumenants: In vitro and in vivo studies. BMC Veterinary Research. 2009;**107**:103-108. DOI: 10.1186/1746-6148-5-46

[40] Paz-Silva A, Francisco I, Valero-Coss RO, Cortiñas FJ, Sánchez JA, Francisco R, et al. Ability of the fungus *Duddingtonia flagrans* to adapt to the cyathostomin egg-output by spreading chlamydospores. Veterinary Parasitology. 2011;**30**:277-282. DOI: 10.1016/j.vetpar.2011.02.014

Chapter 4

Using Host Resistance to Control Cotton Parasitic Reniform Nematode

Chunda Feng, Salliana R. Stetina and John E. Erpelding

Abstract

Cotton (*Gossypium hirsutum*) is the primary source of natural fiber for the textile industry worldwide. The US is a leading cotton producer and the largest exporter for the international cotton market, representing about US$7 billion annually. Reniform nematode (RN, *Rotylenchulus reniformis*) is a major pest for US cotton production. Annual seedcotton yield losses associated with RN are estimated at 1% representing approximately US$100 M loss in production. In the major cotton-producing states of Alabama, Louisiana, and Mississippi, RN has become the most important pest problem. Several approaches are required for RN management. Nematicides are effective in providing protection for cotton seedling development to enhance plant vigor and reduce yield losses, but the RN population will dramatically rebound during the cotton growing season. Rotation with non-host crops will reduce RN populations, but long rotational cycles are required to suppress the rapid recovery of the population. Growing resistant cultivars would be the most effective and sustainable strategy for long-term RN management. However, RN resistance was not found in the widely grown tetraploid upland cotton, thus hindering the rapid development of resistance cultivars. Several Sea Island cottons (*G. barbadense*) highly resistant to RN have been used to develop resistant upland cotton varieties. RN resistance was frequently observed in diploid *Gossypium* species. Our research focuses on introgression of RN resistance from diploid *Gossypium* species to upland cotton, understanding the genetics of resistance to enhance genetic diversity and developing genomic tools that can be applied for studying the genetics of resistance and for marker-assisted breeding.

Keywords: cotton, germplasm, reniform nematode, resistance, pest management, wide hybridization

1. Introduction

The plant-parasitic reniform nematode (RN, *Rotylenchulus reniformis* Linford and Oliveira) is a yield-limiting factor for upland cotton (*Gossypium hirsutum*) production in the US [1]. RN has been found in 13 states (from the East Coast to Texas) representing the upland cotton growing belt of the US, and the number of counties where RN is present has rapidly increased [2]. According to the Cotton Disease Loss Estimate

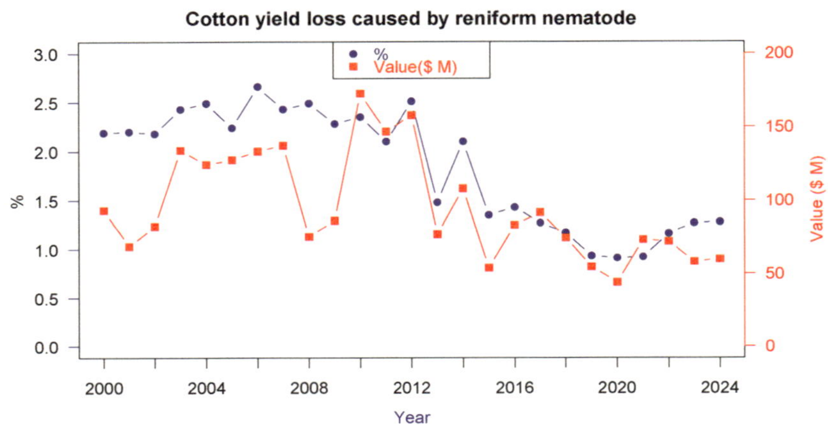

Figure 1.
Estimated percentages and values of annual US cotton production losses attributed to reniform nematode from 2000 to 2024.

Committee reports (https://www.cotton.org/beltwide/proceedings and https://cropprotectionnetwork.org/), annual seedcotton yield losses caused by reniform nematode ranged from 0.91 to 2.66% from 2000 to 2024, equivalent to values of $43.94–$172.65 M (**Figure 1**), with an average loss of $95.60 million per year, and a total of $2.39 billion in the past 25 years, excluding additional costs related to RN management. In the states of Alabama, Louisiana, and Mississippi, RN has replaced root-knot nematode (*Meloidogyne incognita*) as the major nematode pest of cotton [1], and yield losses were estimated from 5 to 9% in these states [3], which were much higher than the nationwide average. In some RN infested fields, yield losses were considerably higher. For example, the average yield loss of seven cultivars was 50% compared to the same cultivars grown in an adjacent non-infested field [4].

2. *Rotylenchulus reniformis*: host range, biology and distribution in soil

2.1 Host plants

RN was first reported infecting roots of cowpea plants grown in pineapple fields in Hawaii during 1940 [5]. In the same year, RN was observed from cotton plants grown in Georgia [6]. RN can infect roots of 314 plant species distributed in 77 families, including some important crops, such as cotton, soybean, cowpea, sweet potato, tomato, and numerous vegetables [7]. Many weed species commonly found in fields of these crops can also be infected [8] and can influence RN management. The feeding of nematodes on the cotton plant will damage the root system, interfering with the uptake of water and nutrients from the soil, which will result in plant stunting, fruit abortion, delayed maturity, and reductions in seedcotton yield, boll size, and lint percentage [9–11]. Seedling death is common under high infestation levels, and these poor stands can result in greater weed competition. Nematode-disease complex is another concern. The wounds resulting from RN feeding increase the plant's vulnerability to soilborne diseases, such as Fusarium wilt and Verticillium wilt. The incidences of Fusarium wilt in wilt-susceptible varieties were 81.4% when RN was present, but only 10% when the nematode was absent [12].

2.2 RN life cycle

The short life cycle of *R. reniformis* makes it difficult to manage the RN population. The egg-to-egg life cycle is about 17–29 days under favorable environmental conditions, and five to seven generations can be produced during a single cotton growing season [1]. Eggs start to hatch about 8 days after deposition. The first-stage juveniles (J1) molt inside the eggs to produce the second-stage juveniles (J2). After three molts, the juveniles develop into young adults with about equal numbers of males and females after 10–14 days (**Figure 2a**). The male nematodes do not infect roots of the host plant and remain in soil. Female vermiform nematodes penetrate the root cortex of the host plant, and the anterior part of the body reaches the endodermal and pericycle cells, whereas the posterior part remains outside the root (**Figure 2b**). The female nematode modifies the host cells at the feeding site to form a syncytium, which is the permanent and sole nutrient source for development and reproduction [13, 14]. The posterior portion of the body swells and forms a characteristic kidney shape (**Figure 2c**). When the gonads reach maturity, the female nematodes lay eggs in a gelatinous matrix (**Figure 2c**) with about 60 but could be up to 200 eggs, approximately 7 days after infection. This high reproduction rate will also influence pest management.

2.3 RN spatial distribution in soil

RN has been observed in many soil types [1, 15]. It is not clear if soil texture has an impact on the distribution of RN. In Texas, RN was frequently found in finely textured soils but was less common in soils with greater than 40% sand content [16]. The population densities of RN in South Carolina soils were correlated to the percentages of sand and silt in the soil until the observed sand content was greater than 60%, resulting in a greater decline in the population density [17]. In contrast, no correlation was observed between RN population densities and soil texture for evaluations conducted in Arkansas, Louisiana, and Texas [18].

Different tillage and crop sequence systems may impact RN population densities and distribution in the soil profile [19]. Holguin et al. reported that the highest population densities occurred at 15–30 cm deep after a cotton crop, but after a non-host crop, higher population densities were recorded deeper in the soil profile [17]. Robinson et al. reported that nematodes were found below 100 cm in about half of the fields investigated, and often more than half the populations were below 30 cm in the soil profile; while in other fields, nematodes were found only in the top 45 cm with the greatest densities occurring in the top 15 cm of the soil profile [18]. The ability of this nematode to survive deep in the soil profile is another factor hindering pest management strategies.

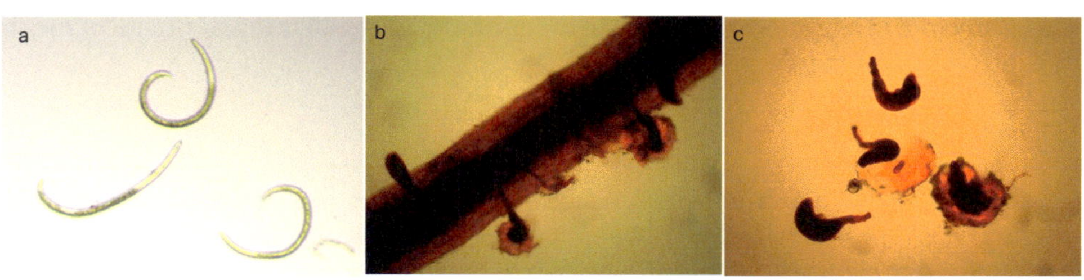

Figure 2.
Immature and mature Rotylenchulus reniformis. *a. vermiform nematodes; b.* R. reniformis *feeding on cotton roots; c. Four mature* R. reniformis *and one egg.*

3. Pest management strategies for RN

3.1 Nematicides

Application of chemical nematicides is the most widely used control strategy. Soil fumigation, in-furrow application, and seed treatment are common methods for the application of nematicides. Nematicide applications have been shown to reduce RN populations and increase seedcotton yields [20]. However, the efficacy of the nematicide may vary due to soil type and environmental conditions during the growing season. Nematicides used for soil fumigation or application in plant furrow could control nematodes in the upper 30–45 cm of soil, but nematodes below this depth can escape the chemical treatment, and the nematode population can dramatically rebound during the growing season, resulting in yield losses [18, 19]. A limited number of nematicides are available for cotton production and the applications may not be profitable [21, 22]. There are also human health and environmental concerns with the use of chemical nematicides.

Sustainable nematicides are alternatives for chemical nematicides that can reduce the environmental impact. Plant essential oils can be used as nematicides for various plant-parasitic nematodes, and the essential oils from *Majorana hortensis*, *M. spicata*, and *Thymus vulgaris* have shown 100% mortality for *R. reniformis* [23]. The antimicrobial and insecticidal functions of chemicals 1,3,4-oxadiazoles have been studied for medical and agricultural uses [24]. Cyprocide (1,3,4-oxadiazole thioether) is bioactivated into a lethal reactive electrophilic metabolite by specific nematode cytochrome P450 enzymes, and thus can selectively kill nematodes, including diverse species of plant-parasitic nematodes [25]. Although these sustainable nematicides have a minimum environmental impact, the costs could limit their use for RN management in cotton.

3.2 Biological control

Two fungal strains (ARF and *Pochonia chlamydosporia*) recovered from RN infested soils in Arkansas were found to be nematophagous [26, 27]. The ARF strain was similar to a previously reported ARF 18 isolate that parasitized soybean cyst nematode (*Heterodera glycines*) [28]. Several isolates of *Pochonia chlamydosporia* could significantly reduce RN numbers on cotton roots and in the soil [27]. *Bacillus firmus* GB-126 and *Paecilomyces lilacinus* 251, applied separately or concomitantly, were shown to reduce the number of eggs and vermiform female nematodes in the soil with seedcotton yields for these treatments similar to the chemical nematicide aldicarb treatment [29]. The infectious bacteria in the genus *Pasteuria* can be used for cotton seed treatment with an efficacy comparable to chemical nematicides [30]. These biological control agents are currently not commercially available as a practical means for controlling *R. reniformis*.

3.3 Crop rotation

Crop rotation with non-host crops, such as corn and peanuts, or with resistant host cultivars, was reported to reduce RN populations [31]; however, long rotational cycles were required to significantly reduce the population to have an economic benefit. RN can survive for at least 2 years in dry soil in an anhydrobiosis manner without a host plant [32], and the RN population could recover in one cotton growing season [19]. Moreover, crop rotation is not always feasible due to economic and resource constraints.

3.4 Resistant cotton cultivars

Growing resistant cultivars or combining approaches of resistant cultivars and nematicide application have been shown to be effective for RN management [1, 33, 34]. Growing commercial resistant cotton cultivars could dramatically reduce the RN populations, and achieve higher yield compared to the susceptible cultivar, and the yield could be further increased with the integration of nematicide management [34]. Singh et al. reported that growing resistant cultivars reduced the RN population by 38% [35]. Using resistant cotton cultivars would be the most economical and effective approach for RN management, and developing upland cotton cultivars with RN resistance is a common goal for cotton breeding programs.

4. Breeding RN resistant upland cotton cultivars

The *Gossypium* genus consists of 55 species, including seven tetraploid (genomes AD1 to AD7) and 48 diploid species (genome groups A to G, and K) [36]. Only four species, including two tetraploids, *G. hirsutum* (upland cotton) and *G. barbadense* (sea island cotton), and two diploids, *G. arboreum* and *G. herbaceum*, are cultivated, with *G. hirsutum* and *G. barbadense* accounting for 95 and 3% of the world cotton production and 97 and 3% of the US cotton production. Based on the potential usages for genetic improvement of the two tetraploid cultigens, the exotic cotton genetic resource comprises in primary germplasm pool (all seven tetraploid species that can cross with cultivated tetraploid species and produce fertile progenies), secondary germplasm pool (A, B, D, F genome species whose chromosomes have reasonably high homoeology to either the A subgenome or the D subgenome of the tetraploid AD species), and tertiary germplasm pool (C, E, G, K genome species whose chromosomes have limited homoeology to the two subgenomes of the tetraploid AD species) [37].

4.1 Screening cotton germplasm accessions for RN resistance

Upland cotton accounts for 97% of US cotton production (USDA-ERS, 2024), and more than 7000 accessions are maintained in the USDA-GRIN upland cotton germplasm collection. Identifying sources of resistance from this collection would be highly desirable for the rapid development of resistant cultivars. The collection has been extensively evaluated [9, 38–41]. Yik and Birchfield identified two accessions, Marie Galante 893 (PI 529860) collected from Haiti and Marie Galante 903 (PI 529864) collected from Cuba that showed RN resistance and one moderately resistant accession, Marie Galante 874 (PI 529852), from St. Thomas, the US Virgin Islands, but no resistant cotton cultivars were developed using these accessions [42]. Additionally, these accessions are photoperiod sensitive, limiting their utilization in breeding programs. Robinson et al. evaluated 1866 accessions with six accessions rated as moderately resistant, and three of these accessions were also resistant to root-knot nematode [38]. Weaver et al. screened 1973 accessions of *G. hirsutum* germplasm, none showed high levels of resistance, seven accessions showed lower RN population development than the susceptible control Paymaster 'PM 1218', and only two out of the six previous identified moderate resistant accessions were confirmed resistant in this test, the discrepancy may result from different nematode populations and/or controls were used [41]. Several breeding lines have been developed from RN resistant upland cotton germplasm, which reduced the RN population to one-half or reduced yield losses to RN by 33% compared to a susceptible cultivar [43, 44]. However, because of the lower level of RN resistance associated with upland cotton germplasm, breeding programs have not extensively utilized these resistant sources for the development of commercial cultivars.

G. barbadense is another commercially cultivated cotton species. Cultivars of the species are grown for their high-quality fiber, but cottonseed yields are lower than upland cotton, and fewer acres are planted. More than 1800 accessions are maintained in the USDA-GRIN *G. barbadense* germplasm collection. This species is also a tetraploid and can be crossed with upland cotton to produce fertile hybrids; thus, the collection was evaluated for RN resistance. Yik and Birchfield evaluated six accessions, and TX 110 (PI 163608) was rated as highly resistant, suggesting useful sources of RN resistance are present in the collection [42]. Two accessions, TX-1347 and TX-1348, were rated as moderately resistant [45]. A more extensive evaluation was conducted by Robinson et al. [38]. From the 907 accessions evaluated, five accessions were rated as resistant and 17 accessions rated as moderately resistant. Accession GB 713 (PI 608139) showed the highest level of resistance, but TX 110 was rated as moderately resistant for this study [38]. Photoperiod sensitivity is commonly observed for *G. barbadense* accessions, and hybrid breakdown has been reported for crosses between *G. barbadense* and upland cotton, thus, additional resources would be required to introgress RN resistance from other *G. barbadense* accessions.

More than 2200 accessions for 33 cotton diploid species are also maintained in the USDA-GRIN cotton germplasm collection [46]. Yik and Birchfield evaluated 32 accessions representing 19 diploid species. The *G. longicalyx* accessions were rated as immune, whereas resistant or moderately resistant accessions were identified from the *G. somalense*, *G. stocksii*, *G. raimondii*, *G. arboreum*, and *G. herbaceum* species included in this study [42]. The diploid species *G. aridum* may also be a source of RN resistance [47]. The two diploid species *G. arboreum* and *G. herbaceum* were once widely cultivated in Asia, and more extensive evaluations have been conducted for these species. Most of the accessions for the two species are photoperiod-insensitive, which aids in the evaluation and breeding of these accessions in temperate regions. More than 1800 accessions for *G. arboreum* and 160 for *G. herbaceum* are maintained in the germplasm collection [46]. RN resistance was more frequently observed for *G. arboreum* accessions with 26 rated as resistant and 102 as moderately resistant [37, 42, 48]. For *G. herbaceum*, four accessions were rated as resistant and 24 accessions as moderately resistant [42, 49]. Although transferring resistance from these species to upland cotton is more difficult, novel sources of RN resistance may be present in the diploid species.

4.2 Genetics of RN resistance

Understanding the genetic basis of resistance is critical for breeding cotton cultivars and will aid in the introgression of resistance from related cotton species; however, few studies have evaluated the genetics of resistance for tetraploid cotton accessions. The inheritance of RN resistance for upland cotton was evaluated by analyzing the generation means of populations developed by crossing the susceptible cultivar 'Deltapine 41' and three cultivars, La RN-910, Auburn (Aub) 612-RNR, M 019-RNR, reported to be resistant, and data suggested complex inheritance of resistance [50]. These findings may have resulted from the low level of resistance associated with the parents; nevertheless, it is likely that the multiple genes with minor effects may be associated with resistance for upland cotton. The RN resistance associated with the *G. barbadense* line GB 713 was controlled by three QTL, two QTL (Ren^{barb1} and Ren^{barb2}) were mapped to chromosome AD_ch21_Dt.11, and the third

QTL (*Ren*^{barb3}) was mapped to chromosome AD_ch18_Dt.13 [51]. These QTL were further mapped to a 17.7 MB interval (36.5–54.2 MB) on AD_ch21_Dt.11 and a 1.8 MB interval (5.9–7.7 MB) on AD_ch18_Dt.13 [52]. Most of the resistance was associated with QTL *Ren*^{barb2} and the presence of QTL *Ren*^{barb3} was required to recover the high level of resistance characteristic of GB 713.

For the cotton diploid species *G. longicalyx*, RN resistance was controlled by one dominant gene *Ren*^{lon}, which was mapped on *G. longicalyx* chromosome 11 [53, 54]. The resistance QTL *Ren*^{ari} from *G. aridum* introgressed into upland cotton (*G. hirsutum* x *G. aridum*) was mapped to the tetraploid chromosome AD_ch21_Dt.11 [47]. For *G. arboreum*, RN resistance was controlled by a single recessive gene for the moderately resistant accession PI 529728 (A2-100) [55], and by two recessive genes for the highly resistant accessions PI 529740 (A2-113) and PI 417895 (A2-87) [56, 57]. The two QTL controlling resistance for PI 417895 have been mapped on chromosomes 10 and 12, and disease resistance genes have been identified in these regions [58]. Using a genome-wide association study approach, 15 significant SNPs associated with RN resistance were identified in a panel of 246 *G. arboreum* accessions, and these SNPs showed additive effects for RN resistance [59]. Eight SNPs identified from a genome-wide association study were linked with resistance in *G. herbaceum* [49]. These studies suggest genetic diversity for RN resistance within the *G. arboreum* and *G. herbaceum* germplasm collections. Transcriptome analysis from several *Gossypium* species revealed differentially expressed genes associated with RN resistance, including disease resistance genes [60, 61]. The application of genomic tools will expedite the genetic dissection of RN resistance for *Gossypium* and facilitate introgression of resistance to upland cotton.

4.3 Developing upland cotton varieties using *G. barbadense* resistance

Multiple upland cotton varieties with improved RN resistance have been developed and released using *G. barbadense* resistance. Using TX 110 and a root-knot nematode resistant *G. hirsutum* line M315 RNR (PI 592514) as parents, two upland cotton lines, TAM RKRNR-9 (PI 662039) and TAM RKRNR-12 (PI 662040), were developed that suppress reniform nematode reproduction by 40–70% and reduce root-knot nematode reproduction by more than 90% [62]. Multiple resistant lines were developed using GB 713 as the source of RN resistance. Three lines, M713Ren1 (PI 665928), M713Ren2 (PI 665929), and M713Ren5 (PI 665930), developed in Mississippi, showed approximately 90% suppression in reniform nematode egg production [63]. The lines BARBREN-713 (PI 671965) and BARBREN-713-32 (PI 701076) developed in Texas suppressed nematode egg production by 74–92% [64, 65]. These GB 713 lines have been used to breed commercial cotton cultivars with RN resistance; however, relying on a single source of resistance could contribute to shifts in the nematode population and the loss of resistance.

4.4 Developing upland cotton varieties using resistance from diploid *Gossypium* species

Crossing diploid species with upland cotton to obtain hybrid seeds is rarely successful. Ovule rescue has been used to recover hybrid plants from these wide hybridizations [66, 67]. The triploid plants that are recovered are typically sterile and are treated with colchicine to double the chromosome number to generate hexaploid plants, which can be crossed with upland cotton or serve as bridging lines to cross with diploid *Gossypium* species [68].

Two upland cotton lines LONREN-1 (PI 669509) and LONREN-2 (PI 669510) were developed using bridging lines (*G. hirsutum* x *G. longicalyx*) and (*G. hirsutum* x *G. herbaceum*) to introgress RN resistance from *G. longicalyx* [54, 69, 70]. These lines were incorporated into many breeding programs; however, plant stunting was commonly observed in breeding lines derived from this source of resistance. Resistance was shown to be associated with a hypersensitive reaction under high nematode pressure, and severe root necrosis and plant stunting were reported [71], thus eliminating the use of this resistance source in commercial cotton breeding programs.

G. hirsutum cultivars have been crossed with several diploid species, including *G. herbaceum* (A1), *G. arboreum* (A2), *G. thurberi* (D1), *G. aridum* (D4), *G. raimondii* (D5), and *G. longicalyx* (F1) to generate additional hexaploid breeding lines. Triploid F1 plants have been obtained through ovule culture [66, 67] or from hybrid seeds harvested in vivo. Abnormal growth was commonly observed for seedling generated from ovule culture reducing the success rate, and some plants showed poor root growth that would require grafting to recover healthy plants. Triploid plants were male and female sterile. The meristematic or lateral buds of triploid plants were treated with 0.2% colchicine for 24 h for chromosome doubling to recover fertility. Several hexaploid lines have been obtained (**Figure 3**). These hexaploid plants can be crossed with upland cotton cultivars to recover the upland cotton phenotype or be used as bridging lines in crosses with other diploid cotton accessions. The hexaploid (*G. hirsutum* x *G. aridum*) bridging line was used to introgress RN resistance from *G. arboreum* and *G. aridum* into upland cotton [47, 72]. So far, no resistant upland cotton lines have been developed using this hexaploid, and these bridging lines are no longer available. Newly developed hexaploid lines are crossed with selected diploid genotypes to introduce resistance to upland cotton.

Autotetraploid *G. arboreum* lines (AAAA) and synthetic allotetraploid (AADD) lines, which can be crossed with *G. hirsutum*, were also developed for introgression of RN resistance. The *G. arboreum* accessions A2-190 (PI 615699), A2-272 (PI 615766), A2-354 (PI 615848), A2-514 (PI 616008), A2-690 (PI 616184), and A2-737 (PI 616231) were rated as highly resistant to reniform nematode [48] and (R x R) F1 plants were treated with colchicine. The chromosomes of five F1 plants (one each from crosses A2-690 x A2-190, A2-690 x A2-272, A2-737 x A2-190, A2-737 x A2-354, A2-737x A2-514) have been doubled. The derived tetraploid plants have larger and thicker leaves compared to their original diploid counterparts (**Figure 4a**), and flowers are larger and usually sterile (**Figure 4b**), boll shapes are different from

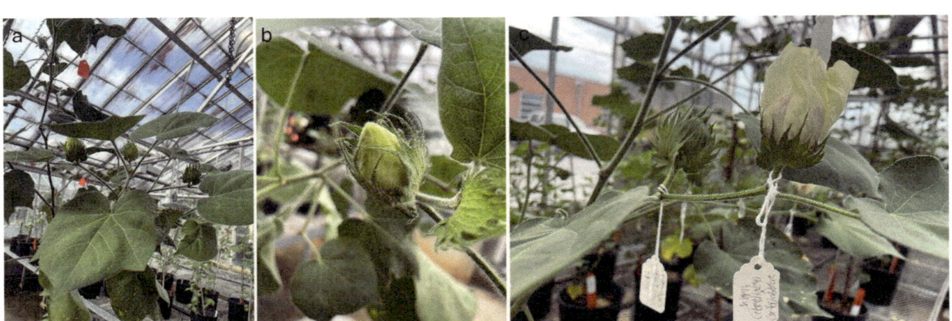

Figure 3.
*A hexaploid plant of (*G. hirsutum x G. raimondii*). a. plant; b. bud; c. flower and boll.*

G. arboreum as well (**Figure 4c**). These plants barely shed pollen but can be crossed with *G. hirsutum* and *G. barbadense* cultivars to produce seeds.

To generate synthetic allotetraploid plants, crosses were made between *G. arboreum* (A2 genome) and the D genome species, *G. aridum* (D4), *G. raimondii* (D5), and *G. trilobum* (D8). A synthetic allotetraploid (A2A2D8D8) plant was obtained through colchicine chromosome doubling (**Figure 5a**). The leaf shape and flowers resemble those of *G. hirsutum*. Flowers are male sterile but can be pollinated with tetraploid cotton cultivars (**Figure 5b**), and the boll shape is different from the parents (**Figure 5c**). Some progenies using this synthetic tetraploid crossed with *G. hirsutum* and *G. barbadense* have been produced for further evaluations.

There are multiple challenges using diploid cotton accessions as a source of RN resistance for the development of upland cotton cultivars. (1) It is difficult to obtain triploid hybrids by crossing tetraploid and diploid cotton species. Triploid plants can be recovered through ovule tissue culture methodology, but the success rate is low, and additional resources and technical expertise are required. (2) The success rate of doubling cotton chromosomes with colchicine was low, which could be as little as 0.1%. (3) Sterility of progenies derived from wide hybridization was highly frequent. Plants of the artificial autotetraploid and allotetraploid, and one hexaploid (AhAhDhDhD5D5) were male sterile. No self-pollinated seeds were obtained from these plants except one boll from an autotetraploid *G. arboreum*. These plants were female fertile and can be pollinated using tetraploid or diploid plants to produce seeds, except for one tetraploid plant of [G. arboreum x 2(ADD)], which was male and female sterile. All triploid hybrids showed female and male sterility, requiring chromosome doubling to recover female fertility. Male fertility can be recovered by

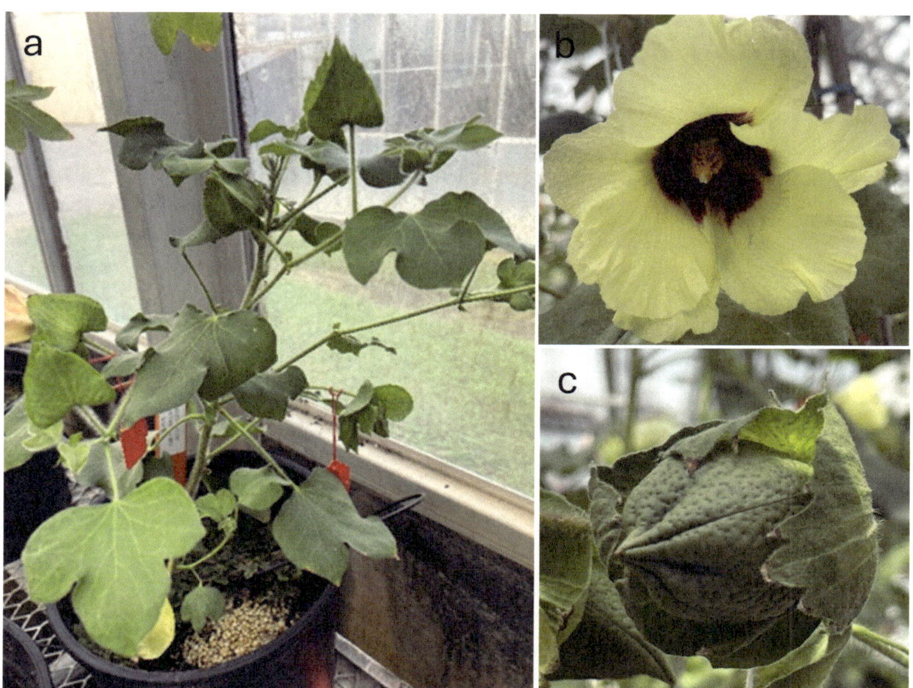

Figure 4.
An autotetraploid plant of (A2-737 x A2-190) F1. a. plant; b. flower; c. boll.

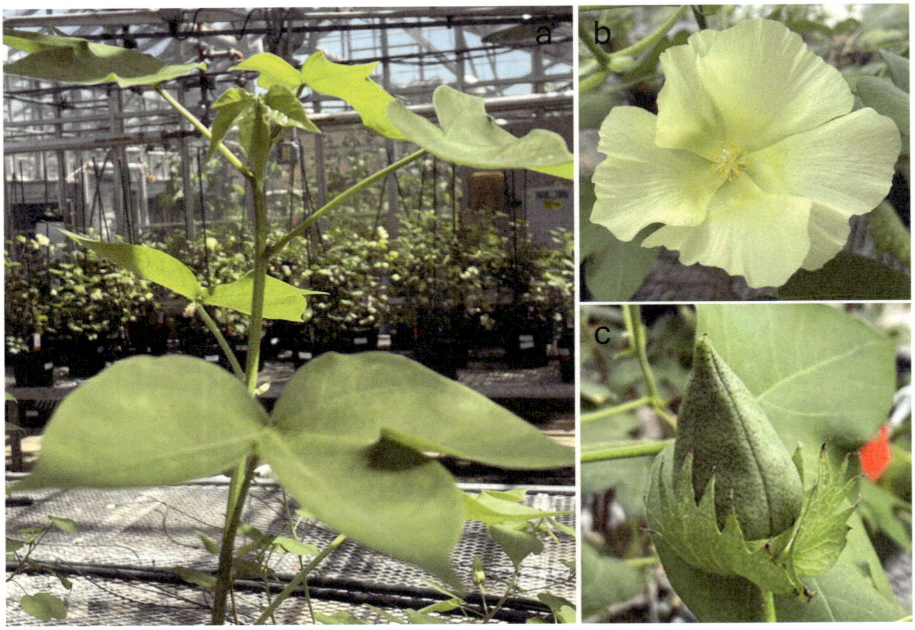

Figure 5.
An allotetraploid plant of (A2A2D8D8). a. plant; b. flower; c. boll.

crossing the hexaploid plants with diploid plants or by backcrossing with *G. hirsutum* cultivars. (4) Dramatic segregation may be observed in the interspecific progenies. RN resistance progeny often showed segregation over multiple generations, even though resistance should have been fixed in previous generations. It is possible that high rates of recombination or chromosomal rearrangements at the site of integration in the *G. hirsutum* genome result in a loss of function for the resistance gene. Alternatively, a lack of recombination between different genomes could result in the elimination of the donor genome. The inherent variability in screening for RN resistance can also impede the recovery of resistant progeny. (5) When RN resistance is controlled by recessive gene(s), as observed for several *G. arboreum* genotypes, large populations are required to recover progenies showing a constant resistant response over multiple generations. Marker-assisted selection will be critical for breeding resistant upland cultivars. However, DNA markers tightly linked to resistance will be essential to recover plants where recombination has occurred between the diploid and tetraploid genomes. Variability in evaluating RN resistance and the ability to evaluate large populations can impact the identification of DNA markers linked to resistance genes.

However, there are many benefits for the utilization of RN resistant diploid germplasm in cotton breeding programs. Narrow genetic diversities among modern upland cotton cultivars have created a bottleneck that has restricted genetic improvement. Introgression of RN resistance from diploid species can capture genetic diversity lacking in upland cultivars. Moreover, resistance to other biotic and abiotic stresses, such as bacterial blight, Fusarium wilt race 4, Verticillium wilt, various viruses, drought, and soil salinity, may be introduced to upland cotton. Moreover, along with increases in fiber yield, fiber quality can be improved as well. Tetraploid progenies derived from *G. arboreum* accessions have premium fiber qualities, especially fiber strength (data not shown). The autotetraploid, allotetraploid, and hexaploid bridging lines will make it possible to introduce RN resistance into upland cotton to increase cotton productivity and profitability for growers.

5. New technologies for RN management

Genome editing offers a promising approach for controlling plant-parasitic nematodes [73]. The RNA interference (RNAi) strategy, through the expression of a putative double-stranded RNA (dsRNA) in the host plant to silence important genes involved in nematode development or parasitism, could ultimately reduce the nematode's ability to infect the host plant and reproduce [74]. This method has been used to improve tolerance to root-knot nematode for cotton [75]. Some genes may facilitate pathogenesis in plant-nematode interactions. Loss of function of these susceptibility genes through CRISPR gene editing may be an alternative strategy for RN management [73, 76]. A better understanding of the genes involved in RN resistance would be required to successfully use these technologies.

Acknowledgements

The authors are grateful to Dr. Fang Bai and Dr. Abdelraheem Abdelraheem for their critical review of the manuscript. Mention of trade names or commercial products in this publication is solely for the purpose of providing specific information and does not imply recommendation or endorsement by the U.S. Department of Agriculture. This research was supported by the U.S. Department of Agriculture, Agricultural Research Service under agreement number 6066-22000-094-000D. USDA is an equal opportunity provider and employer.

Author details

Chunda Feng*, Salliana R. Stetina and John E. Erpelding
USDA, Agricultural Research Service, Crop Genetics Research Unit, Stoneville, MS, USA

*Address all correspondence to: chunda.feng@usda.gov

References

[1] Robinson AF. Reniform in U.S. cotton: When, where, why, and some remedies. Annual Review of Phytopathology. 2007;**45**:263-288

[2] Faske TR, Watson T, Desaeger J, Duffeck MR, Eisenback J, Floyd C, et al. Summarized distribution of the reniform nematode, *Rotylenchulus reniformis*, in field crops in the United States. Plant Health Progress. 2024;**25**(4):506-508

[3] Blasingame D. 2005 cotton disease loss estimate. In: Proceedings of the Beltwide Cotton Conferences. San Antonio, TX: National Cotton Council; 2006. pp. 155-157

[4] Dyer DR, Groover W, Lawrence KS. Yield loss of cotton cultivars due to *Rotylenchulus reniformis* and the added benefit of a nematicide. Plant Health Progress. 2020;**21**(2):113-118

[5] Linford MB, Oliveira JM. *Rotylenchulus reniformis*, nov. gen., n. sp., a nematode parasite of roots. Proceedings of the Helminthological Society of Washington. 1940;7:35-42

[6] Smith AL. Distribution and relation of meadow nematode, *Pratylenchus pratensis* to fusarium wilt of cotton in Georgia. Phytopathology. 1940;**30**:710

[7] Robinson AF, Inserra RN, Caswell-Chen EP, Vovlas N, Troccoli A. *Rotylenchulus* species: Identification, distribution, host ranges, and crop plant resistance. Nematropica. 1997:127-180

[8] Lawrence KS. Weed hosts for *Rotylenchulus reniformis* in cotton fields rotated with corn in the southeast of the United States. Nematropica. 2008;**38**(1):13-22

[9] Cook CG, Robinson AF, Namken LN. Tolerance to *Rotylenchulus reniformis* and resistance to *Meloidogyne incognita* race 3 in high-yielding breeding lines of upland cotton. Journal of Nematology. 1997;**29**(3):322-328

[10] Jones JE, Newsom LD, Finley EL. Effect of the reniform nematode on yield, plant characters, and fiber properties of upland cotton. Agronomy Journal. 1959;**51**(6):353-356

[11] Koenning SR, Wrather JA, Kirkpatrick TL, Walker NR, Starr JL, Mueller JD. Plant-parasitic nematodes attacking cotton in the United States: Old and emerging production challenges. Plant Disease. 2004;**88**(2):100-113

[12] MacGowan JB. The reniform nematode. Nematology Circular. 1977;**32**:1-2

[13] Agudelo P, Robbins RT, Kim KS, Stewart JM. Histological changes in *Gossypium hirsutum* associated with reduced reproduction of *Rotylenchulus reniformis*. Journal of Nematology. 2005;**37**(2):185-189

[14] Carter WW. Resistance and resistant reaction of *Gossypium arboreum* to the reniform nematode, *Rotylenchulus reniformis*. Journal of Nematology. 1981;**13**(3):368-374

[15] Gazaway WS, McLean KS. A Survey of Plant-Parasitic Nematodes Associated with Cotton in Alabama. 2003;7:1

[16] Starr JL, Heald CM, Robinson AF, Smith RG, Krausz JP. *Meloidogyne incognita* and *Rotylenchulus reniformis* and associated soil textures from some cotton production areas of Texas. Journal of Nematology. 1993;**25**(4S):895-899

[17] Holguin CM, Gerard P, Mueller JD, Khalilian A, Agudelo P. Spatial distribution of reniform nematode in cotton as influenced by soil texture and crop rotations. Phytopathology. 2015;**105**(5):674-683

[18] Robinson AF, Cook CG, Kirkpatrick TL, McGawley EC, Overstreet C, Padgett B. Vertical distribution of the reniform nematode in the upper 1.5 meters of soil on nine farms in Arkansas, Louisiana, and Texas. In: Proceeding of the Beltwide Cotton Conferences. 2000. p. 564. Available from: https://www.cotton.org/beltwide/proceedings/2000/abstracts/254.cfm

[19] Westphal A, Smart JR. Depth distribution of *Rotylenchulus reniformis* under different tillage and crop sequence systems. Phytopathology. 2003;**93**(9):1182-1189

[20] Lawaju BR, Chetri P, Bhandari G, Lawrence K. Nematicide and cotton variety combinations for managing reniform nematodes in North Alabama, 2024. Plant Health Progress. 2024. Available from: https://apsjournals.apsnet.org/doi/abs/10.1094/PHP-02-25-0039-PDMR

[21] Grabau ZJ, Liu C, Schumacher LA, Small IM, Wright DL. In-furrow fluopyram nematicide efficacy for *Rotylenchulus reniformis* management in cotton production. Crop Protection. 2021;**140**:105423

[22] Wilson BR, Allen TW, Catchot AL, Krutz LJ, Dodds DM. Determining the profitability of reniform nematode control practices in the Mississippi cotton production system. Plant Health Progress. 2020;**21**(2):105-112

[23] Catani L, Manachini B, Grassi E, Guidi L, Semprucci F. Essential oils as nematicides in plant protection—A review. Plants. 2023;**12**(6):1418

[24] Luczynski M, Kudelko A. Synthesis and biological activity of 1,3,4-oxadiazoles used in medicine and agriculture. Applied Sciences. 2022;**12**(8):3756

[25] Knox J, Burns AR, Cooke B, Cammalleri SR, Kitner M, Ching J, et al. Cyprocide selectively kills nematodes via cytochrome P450 bioactivation. Nature Communications. 2024;**15**(1):5529

[26] Wang K, Riggs RD, Crippen D. Suppression of *Rotylenchulus reniformis* on cotton by the nematophagous fungus ARF. Journal of Nematology. 2004;**36**(2):186-191

[27] Wang K, Riggs RD, Crippen D. Isolation, selection, and efficacy of *Pochonia chlamydosporia* for control of *Rotylenchulus reniformis* on cotton. Phytopathology. 2005;**95**(8):890-893

[28] Kim DG, Riggs RD. Characteristics and efficacy of a sterile Hyphomycete (ARF18), a new biocontrol agent for *Heterodera glycines* and other nematodes. Journal of Nematology. 1991;**23**(3):275-282

[29] Castillo JD, Lawrence KS, Kloepper JW. Biocontrol of the reniform nematode by *Bacillus firmus* GB-126 and *Paecilomyces lilacinus* 251 on cotton. Plant Disease. 2013;**97**(7):967-976

[30] Schmidt LM, Hewlett TE, Green A, Simmons LJ, Kelley K, Doroh M, et al. Molecular and morphological characterization and biological control capabilities of a Pasteuria ssp. parasitizing Rotylenchulus reniformis, the Reniform nematode. Journal of Nematology. 2010;**42**(3):207-217

[31] Stetina SR, Young LD, Pettigrew WT, Bruns HA. Effect of corn-cotton

rotations on reniform nematode populations and crop yield. Nematropica. 2007;**37**:237-248

[32] Radewald JD, Takeshita G. Desiccation studies on five species of plant-parasitic nematodes of Hawaii. Phytopathology. 1964;**54**:903-904

[33] Lahlali R, Banu G, Mokrini F, Ibrahim DSS, Belabess Z. Nematode problems in cotton and their sustainable management. In: Nematode Diseases of Crops and their Sustainable Management. San Diego, CA, USA: Elsevier; 2023. pp. 531-564. Available from: https://linkinghub.elsevier.com/retrieve/pii/B9780323912266000043

[34] Turner AK, Graham SH, Potnis N, Brown SM, Donald P, Lawrence KS. Evaluation of *Meloidogyne incognita* and *Rotylenchulus reniformis* nematode-resistant cotton cultivars with supplemental Corteva Agriscience nematicides. Journal of Nematology. 2023;**55**(1):1-21

[35] Singh B, Chastain D, Reddy KR, Snider J, Krutz LJ, Stetina S, et al. Agronomic characterization of cotton genotypes susceptible and resistant to reniform nematode in the United States Midsouth. Agronomy Journal. 2021;**113**(5):4280-4291

[36] Wang K, Wendel JF, Hua J. Designations for individual genomes and chromosomes in Gossypium. Journal of Cotton Research. 2018;**1**(1):3

[37] Stewart JM, Feng C. Utilization of exotic cotton germplasm resources to increase genetic diversity. In: Proceeding of World Cotton Research Conference. Cape Town, South Africa: International Cotton Advisory Committee; 2003. pp. 194-197

[38] Robinson AF, Bridges AC, Percival AE. New sources of resistance to the reniform (*Rotylenchulus reniformis* Linford and Oliveira) and root-knot (*Meloidogyne incognita* (Kofoid & White) Chitwood) nematode in upland (*Gossypium hirsutum* L.) and Sea Island (*G. Barbadense L.*) cotton. The Journal of Cotton Science. 2004;**8**(3):191-197

[39] Robinson AF, Percival AE. Resistance to Meloidogyne incognita race 3 and Rotylenchulus reniformis in wild accessions of Gossypium hirsutum and *G. barbadense* from Mexico. The Journal of Nematology. 1997;**29**(4S):746

[40] Usery SR Jr, Lawrence KS, Lawrence GW, Burmester CH. Evaluation of cotton cultivars for resistance and tolerance to *Rotylenchulus reniformis*. Nematropica. 2005;**35**:121-134

[41] Weaver DB, Lawrence KS, van Santen E. Reniform nematode resistance in upland cotton germplasm. Crop Science. 2007;**47**(1):19-24

[42] Yik CP, Birchfield W. Resistant germplasm in Gossypium species and related plants to *Rotylenchulus reniformis*. Journal of Nematology. 1984;**16**(2):146-153

[43] Cook CG, Robinson AF. Registration of RN96425, RN96527, and RN96625-1 nematode-resistant cotton germplasm lines. Crop Science. 2005;**45**(4):1667-1668

[44] McCarty JC, Jenkins JN, Wubben MJ, Hayes RW, LaFoe JM II. Registration of three germplasm lines of cotton derived from *Gossypium hirsutum* L. accession T2468 with moderate resistance to the reniform nematode. Journal of Plant Registrations. 2012;**6**(1):85-87

[45] Robinson AF, Percival AE. Resistance to *Meloidogyne incognita* race 3 and *Rotylenchulus reniformis* in wild accessions of *Gossypium hirsutum* and *G. Barbadense* from Mexico. Journal of Nematology. 1997;**29**(4S):746-755

[46] Percy RG, Frelichowski JE, Arnold MD, Campbell TB, Dever JK, Fang DD, et al. The U.S. National Cotton Germplasm Collection – Its contents, preservation, characterization, and evaluation. In: World Cotton Germplasm Resources. London, UK: IntechOpen; 2014. Available from: https://www.intechopen.com/chapters/47112

[47] Romano GB, Sacks EJ, Stetina SR, Robinson AF, Fang DD, Gutierrez OA, et al. Identification and genomic location of a reniform nematode (*Rotylenchulus reniformis*) resistance locus (Ren^{ari}) introgressed from *Gossypium aridum* into upland cotton (*G. Hirsutum*). Theoretical and Applied Genetics. 2009;**120**(1):139-150

[48] Stetina SR, Erpelding JE. *Gossypium arboreum* accessions resistant to *Rotylenchulus reniformis*. Journal of Nematology. 2016;**48**(4):223-230

[49] Feng C, Stetina SR, Erpelding JE. Genome-wide association study of the resistance of *Gossypium herbaceum* to reniform nematode. Euphytica. 2025;**221**

[50] Muhammad N, Jones JE. Genetics of resistance to reniform nematode in upland cotton. Crop Science. 1990;**30**(1):13-16

[51] Gutiérrez OA, Robinson AF, Jenkins JN, McCarty JC, Wubben MJ, Callahan FE, et al. Identification of QTL regions and SSR markers associated with resistance to reniform nematode in *Gossypium barbadense L.* accession GB713. Theoretical and Applied Genetics. 2011;**122**(2):271-280

[52] Perkin LC, Bell A, Hinze LL, Suh CPC, Arick MA, Peterson DG, et al. Genome assembly of two nematode-resistant cotton lines (*Gossypium hirsutum L.*). G3 (Bethesda). 2021;**11**(11):jkab276

[53] Dighe ND, Robinson AF, Bell AA, Menz MA, Cantrell RG, Stelly DM. Linkage mapping of resistance to reniform nematode in cotton following introgression from *Gossypium longicalyx* (hutch. & lee). Crop Science. 2009;**49**(4):1151-1164

[54] Robinson AF, Bell AA, Dighe ND, Menz MA, Nichols RL, Stelly DM. Introgression of resistance to nematode *Rotylenchulus reniformis* into upland cotton (*Gossypium hirsutum*) from *Gossypium longicalyx*. Crop Science. 2007;**47**(5):1865-1877

[55] Erpelding JE, Stetina SR. Genetics of reniform nematode resistance in *Gossypium arboreum* germplasm line PI 529728. World Journal of Agricultural Research. 2013;**1**(4):48-53

[56] Erpelding JE, Stetina SR. Genetic characterization of reniform nematode resistance for *Gossypium arboreum* accession PI 417895. Plant Breeding. 2018;**137**(1):81-88

[57] Erpelding JE, Stetina SR. Genetic characterization of *Gossypium arboreum* accession PI 529740 for reniform nematode resistance. Plant Breeding. 2019;**138**(6):871-879

[58] Feng C, Stetina SR, Erpelding JE. Mapping QTLs controlling resistance of *Gossypium arboreum* to reniform nematode. In: ASA-CSSA-SSA International Annual Meeting. San Antonio, TX: ASA-CSSA-SSSA; 2024. p. 160557

[59] Li R, Erpelding JE, Stetina SR. Genome-wide association study of *Gossypium arboreum* resistance to reniform nematode. BMC Genetics. 2018;**19**(1):52

[60] Feng C, Stetina SR, Erpelding JE. Transcriptome analysis of resistant cotton germplasm responding

to reniform nematodes. Plants. 2024;**13**(7):958

[61] Li R, Rashotte AM, Singh NK, Lawrence KS, Weaver DB, Locy RD. Transcriptome analysis of cotton (*Gossypium hirsutum* L.) genotypes that are susceptible, resistant, and hypersensitive to reniform nematode (*Rotylenchulus reniformis*). PLoS One. 2015;**10**(11):e0143261

[62] Starr JL, Smith CW, Ripple K, Zhou E, Nichols RL, Faske TR. Registration of TAM RKRNR-9 and TAM RKRNR-12 germplasm lines of upland cotton resistant to reniform and root-knot nematodes. Journal of Plant Registrations. 2011;**5**(3):393-396

[63] McCarty JC Jr, Jenkins JN, Wubben MJ, Gutierrez OA, Hayes RW, Callahan FE, et al. Registration of three germplasm lines of cotton derived from *Gossypium barbadense* L. accession GB713 with resistance to the reniform nematode. Journal of Plant Registrations. 2013;**7**(2):220-223

[64] Bell AA, Robinson AF, Quintana J, Duke SE, Starr JL, Stelly DM, et al. Registration of BARBREN-713 germplasm line of upland cotton resistant to reniform and root-knot nematodes. Journal of Plant Registrations. 2015;**9**(1):89-93

[65] Bell AA, Robinson AF, Quintana J, Hinze LL, Harris J, Liu J, et al. Registration of eight germplasm lines of upland cotton (*Gossypium hirsutum* L.) resistant to reniform nematodes (*Rotylenchulus reniformis*) with elite agronomic performance. Journal of Plant Registrations. 2023;**17**(3):536-543

[66] Erpelding JE. Selection of Gossypium hirsutum genotypes for interspecific introgression from *G. arboreum* using ovule culture. African Journal of Biotechnology. 2015;**14**(16):1373-1378

[67] Sacks EJ. Ovule rescue efficiency of *Gossypium hirsutum* × *G. arboreum* progeny from field-grown fruit is affected by media composition and antimicrobial compounds. Plant Cell, Tissue and Organ Culture. 2008;**93**(1):15-20

[68] JMcD S. Potential for crop improvement with exotic germplasm and genetic engineering. In: Proceedings of the World Cotton Research Conference-1, Brisbane, Australia, February 14-17, Melborune, Australia. 1995. Available from: https://cir.nii.ac.jp/crid/1573387450255387776

[69] Bell AA, Forest Robinson A, Quintana J, Dighe ND, Menz MA, Stelly DM, et al. Registration of LONREN-1 and LONREN-2 germplasm lines of upland cotton resistant to reniform nematode. Journal of Plant Registrations. 2014;**8**(2):187-190

[70] Bell A, Robinson AF. Development and characteristics of triple species hybrids used to transfer reniform nematode resistance from *Gossypium longicalyx* to *Gossypium hirsutum*. In: Proceeding of the Beltwide Cotton Conferences. San Antonio, TX: National Cotton Council; 2004. pp. 422-426

[71] Nichols RL, Bell AA, Stelly DM, Dighe ND, Robinson AF, Menz MA, et al. Phenotypic and genotypic evaluation of LONREN germplasm. In: Proceeding of the Beltwide Cotton Conferences. New Orleans, Louisiana: National Cotton Council; 2010. pp. 798-799

[72] Sacks EJ, Robinson AF. Introgression of resistance to reniform nematode (*Rotylenchulus reniformis*) into upland cotton (*Gossypium hirsutum*) from *Gossypium arboreum* and a

G. Hirsutum/Gossypium aridum bridging line. Field Crops Research. 2009;**112**(1):1-6

[73] Siddique S, Eves-van Den Akker S. Nematode management through genome editing. In: Sikora RA, Desaeger J, Molendijk L, editors. Integrated Nematode Management: State-of-the-Art and Visions for the Future. 1st ed. UK: CABI; 2021. pp. 408-413. Available from: http://www.cabidigitallibrary.org/doi/10.1079/9781789247541.0057

[74] Dutta SD, Ganguly K, Lim KT. RNAi-based gene silencing in plant-parasitic nematodes: A road toward crop improvements. In: Abd-Elsalam KA, Lim KT, editors. CRISPR and RNAi Systems. Cambridge, MA, USA: Elsevier; 2021. pp. 579-596 (Nanobiotechnology for Plant Protection). Available from: https://www.sciencedirect.com/science/article/pii/B9780128219102000084

[75] Lisei-de-Sá ME, Rodrigues-Silva PL, Morgante CV, de Melo BP, Lourenço-Tessutti IT, Arraes FBM, et al. Pyramiding dsRNAs increases phytonematode tolerance in cotton plants. Planta. 2021;**254**(6):121

[76] Engler JDA, Favery B, Engler G, Abad P. Loss of susceptibility as an alternative for nematode resistance. Current Opinion in Biotechnology. 2005;**16**(2):112-117

Chapter 5

Responses of Tree Tomato (*Solanum betaceum*) Varieties to Root-Knot Nematodes (*Meloidogyne* Spp.)

Waswa Stanlous Juma, Waceke Joyce Wajohi and Nchore Shem Bonuke

Abstract

Tree tomato (*Solanum betaceum* Cav.) is an important fruit in Kenya with growing popularity among farmers and consumers due to potential as an income earner and health benefits. The fruit generate rural income and enhances food and nutritional security. Root-knot nematodes (RKNs) pose a major threat to its production. This study determined responses of six tree tomato varieties (goldmine, ruby red, rothamer and red oratia, red light oratia, and grafted) to RKN infection. Rhizosphere soil and roots from 216 plants were collected. Nematodes were extracted and enumerated from 200 cm^3 of soil and 5 grams of roots using modified Baermann tray method. Under greenhouse, seedlings were inoculated with 2000 J2s per pot replicated four times in completely randomized design. Under field, experiments were established in naturally infested field at Kenyatta University and treatments replicated thrice in randomized complete block design. BioNematon-treated plots served as absolute control. Data on plant growth and disease parameters were subjected to analysis of variance using SAS software version 9.1. Means were separated using Tukey's Honestly Significant Difference (HSD) at $P \leq 0.05$. Regression and t-test analysis were done to check for relationships between parameters and significant differences between means, respectively. Based on the nematode reproduction factor rated on 0–5 scale, ruby red, rothamer, and red oratia were moderately resistant both in both tests. Red light oratia and grafted tree tomato were moderately resistant in the greenhouse but tolerant in the field. Moderately resistant and tolerant varieties should be promoted to farmers to manage RKNs in tree tomato.

Keywords: tree tomato, root-knot nematodes, food security, nematode reproduction, plant resistance

1. Introduction

Tree tomato also called tamarillo (*Solanum betaceum* CAV.), is a native fruit to the South American Andes and is currently grown worldwide [1, 2]. Production of tree tomato in Kenya was 5111 and 7433 metric tons for years 2014 and 2016, respectively [3]. Apart from trade, the tree tomato fruit is used as fresh fruit juice and in food processing industries. The fruit is rich in vitamins A, B, C, E, calcium, iron, phosphorus, anthocyanin, and antioxidants [4] and therefore important for nutritional security. Anthocyanins present protect the body against diabetes, aging and neurological disorders [4]. The lycopene present keeps off degenerative diseases, improves heart health, and helps the skin's ability to withstand UV radiation [4]. Lycopene is also associated with decreased incidence of several types of cancers, including breast cancer and prostate cancer [5]. Six main varieties of tree tomatoes are grown in Kenya which include goldmine, rothamer, red oratia, ruby red, red light oratia and tree tomato grafted on *Solanum mauritianum* rootstock.

The major challenge facing tree tomato farming in Kenya is infestation by plant-parasitic nematodes (PPN) [6]. Among the PPNs, root-knot nematodes (*Meloidogyne* spp.) are the most serious crop-damaging pest that are polyphagous and are widely distributed in many farming systems [7, 8]. Root-knot nematodes causes root galling which interferes with water and nutrient uptake [9]. In a study conducted in Colombia, *Meloidogyne*, *Helicotylenchus* and *Pratylenchus* were associated with tree tomato cultivation [1].

Root-knot nematodes in tree tomato have been managed through use of chemical nematicides and crop rotation. However, nematicides are harmful to the environment and human health, lose efficacy after prolonged use and are expensive, hence, increasing the cost of production. The use of resistant tree tomato varieties can be the most effective, economical and ecofriendly method of managing RKNs. This study determined the responses of six tree tomato varieties to RKNs under greenhouse and field conditions.

2. Literature review

2.1 Origin and biology of tree tomato

Tree tomato (*Solanum betaceum* Cav.), also known as "tamarillo," belongs to the Solanaceae family that originated from the Andean region of Latin America. Tree tomato is also grown throughout sub-tropical and tropical areas in Colombia, Peru, New Zealand, Haiti, Mexico, Malaysia and Uganda [9]. The name tamarillo was coined in New Zealand [1]. According to the Oxfarm Organic report of 2017 (http:// www.oxfarmorganic.com/our-products/tree-tomato/tips-on-how-to-get-over20kgs-tree-from-tree-tomato-farming/) [10], tree tomatoes were introduced in Kenya by Asians in the late 1800s.

Tree tomato is a perennial plant that grows to a height of about 2–3 m and reaches its maximum yield at 4–5 years [1, 9]. Tree tomatoes produce fruits for up to 10 years [11]. The trees grow between 600 and 3000 m above sea level with optimum growth temperature of 16–20°C, soil pH values of 5.6–7.7, and prefer sandy soils, but the presence of organic matter improves its growth [1]. In developing countries, tree tomato is a subsistence crop cataloged as a marginal species [2], while in Kenya, it is cultivated as a smallholder fruit tree [12].

Tree tomatoes have a very shallow root system that is not very much extensive and grows by forming a single woody trunk at the base and form branches at a height of about 1.5–2 m [11]. It has large simple leaves and produces fragrant flowers with pink-white corolla in clusters of 10–50 hanging on the branches [11]. Flowers are self-pollinated by wind or insects, while the fruits are oval and about 4–8 cm long and 3–5 cm wide although variations do exist [11]. Tamarillo fruits contain very many seeds while the skin color of fruits ranges between yellow, purple and orange and sometimes with longitudinal stripes [11].

2.2 Tree tomato varieties and their production in Kenya

The main varieties of tree tomato grown in Kenya are the goldmine, Inca red, rothamer, solid gold, red oratia, grafted and ruby red (https://www.crfg.org/pubs/ff/tamarillo.html). All varieties of tree tomato are reported to be affected by plant parasitic nematodes but not unequally [13]. In Kenya, tree tomato is mainly grown in highland areas of Kiambu, Nyeri, Embu, Meru, Nyandarua and many Rift valley regions. The fruit is grown alongside other crops like tea, coffee, vegetable crops, and other fruit crops.

There are about eight cultivars known worldwide: Equatorian orange cultivar fruit is medium orange in color with light orange pulp, creamy in texture and less acidic than the ruby red. It is excellent for eating out of hand and suitable for culinary purposes. Red oratia (**Figure 1**) is a large red fruit cultivar that is oval to round in shape with a sharp acidic flavor. Good quality for eating out of hand and excellent for jams and preserves. Goldmine (**Figure 1**) is a superior cultivar originating in New Zealand, and it was recently introduced in Kenya. It is a very large golden-yellow fruit with golden, highly flavored flesh, less bland than solid gold, but not acidic and has superb eating qualities (https://www.crfg.org/pubs/ff/tamarillo.html).

Ruby red (**Figure 1**) is a large, brilliant red fruit with a dark red pulp that is tart and flavorful. Fair for eating out of hand, but very good for culinary use. When allowed to ripen for one to three weeks after picking, they become less acidic. Inca gold is a yellow-fruited cultivar that is less acidic than the red types. When cooked, the fruit resembles the apricot in flavor while solid gold is a large, oval-shaped fruit with a golden-orange skin in color. The pulp of solid gold fruit is soft, less acidic in flavor than red oatia and generally very good for eating out of hand, with acceptable culinary qualities.

Rothamer (**Figure 1**) on the other hand is a large fruit with bright red skin. The flesh of the fruit is golden-yellow with a sweet flavor and exotic with dark red seeds. The fruit ripens from December to April. It is delicious, eaten out of hand, and a vigorously heavy-bearing plant.

Grafted tree tomato varieties are also grown in Kenya. Grafting is done to improve production, resist pests and diseases, and enhance early maturity and longer lifespan. Grafting of tree tomato is done with a bug weed (*Muthakwa*) scientifically known as *Solanum mauritianum*, a wild tree that naturally grows in any conditions. *Muthakwa* has tap root system and is resistant to *Ralstonia*. The extensive taproot system makes it ideal for improved nutrient intake and efficient water absorption which makes the plant resist drought [14]. Propagation has also been done using cuttings. However, plants produced from cuttings do not grow tall and tend to be bushy [11].

Tree tomatoes are attacked by PPNs, insect pests such as aphids, greenhouse whitefly, tomato worm, thrips, green vegetable bug, fruit flies, snails, and slugs [11]. Fungal diseases include powdery mildews, tomato leaf spot, root rot, and anthracnose. Bacterial diseases that infect tree tomatoes include bacterial canker, bacterial blast and crown canker. Viruses have also been reported to affect tree tomato. They include tomato mosaic virus, cucumber mosaic virus, alfalfa mosaic virus, tomato spotted wilt virus, arabis mosaic virus, tobacco mosaic virus, and tomato aspermy

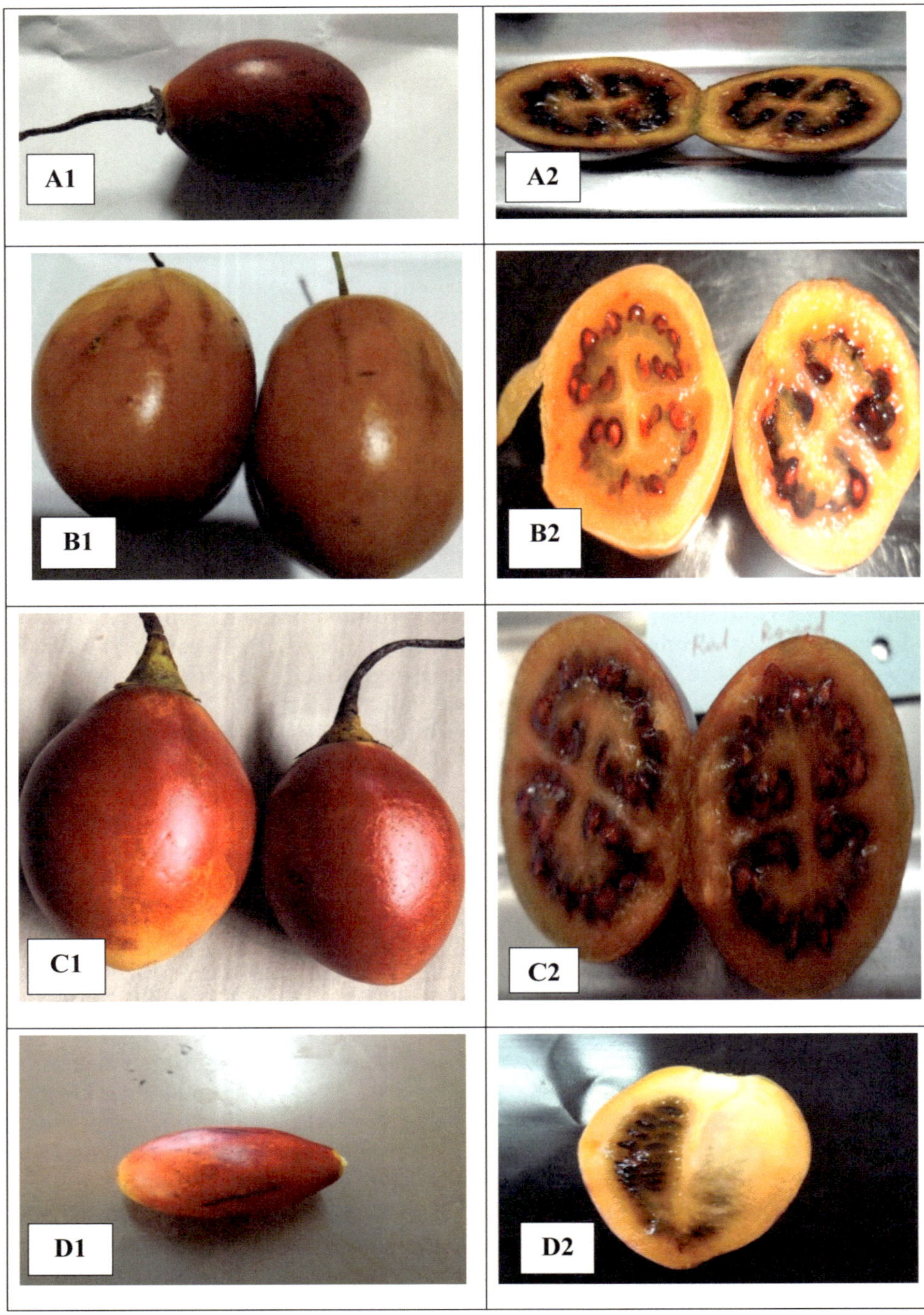

Figure 1.
A1 and A2 = Red oratia whole fruit and transverse section; B1 and B2 = Goldmine whole fruit and transverse section; C1 and C2 = Ruby Red whole fruits and transverse section; D1 and D2 = Rothamer whole fruit and longitudinal section. Source: Own photos from the field in Kiambu and Embu counties, Kenya.

virus [2, 11, 13]. Other production constraints are moisture stress, lack of suitable varieties and certified planting materials, and limited knowledge on appropriate agronomic and post-harvest practices [12].

2.3 Economic importance and health benefits of tree tomato

Tree tomato like other horticultural crops plays a critical role in the economy of developing nations [15]. In 2014, the area, production, and value of tree tomato in Kenya were 619 ha, 5111 tons, and KES.156.3 million, respectively [3] while in 2016 it was 873 ha, 7434 tons, and KES.341.7 million, respectively [16]. The fruit is rich in vitamins A, B, C, E, calcium, iron, phosphorus, and antioxidants. They also contain anthocyanin, which protects the body against diabetes, aging and neurological disorders [4]. The lycopene present keeps off degenerative diseases, improves heart health, and helps the skin's ability to withstand UV radiation [4]. Lycopene is also associated with decreased incidence of several types of cancers, including breast cancer and prostate cancer [5].

3. Materials and methods

Four-week-old seedlings of six tree tomato varieties of Goldmine, Ruby Red, Rothamer, Red Oratia, Red Light Oratia and grafted were planted in the greenhouse in pots containing three kilograms of sterilized soil (2:1, sand:soil mixture) and in the field. The populations of RKN inoculum for resistance screening were multiplied on a susceptible tomato variety (Carl-J). Nematode eggs were extracted by cutting the tomato roots into 1 cm pieces and agitating in 0.5% NaOCl for four minutes [17]. The resultant suspension was washed through 106 and 20 μm sieves with distilled water and incubated. Seedlings in the greenhouse were inoculated with 2000 freshly hatched *Meloidogyne* J2s around the roots seven days after transplanting. Uninoculated plants served as controls. The treatments were labeled and arranged in a completely randomized design with four replicates each at Kenyatta University in the plant sciences greenhouse. The plants were regularly watered as required. In the field, seedlings were planted in a naturally nematode-infested field at Kenyatta University agriculture farm in 3mx3m plots. The treatments were replicated thrice in randomized complete block design, making a total of 18 plots of nematode infestation, each having 12 plants, giving a total of 216 tree tomato plants. The same treatments were applied to nematode-infested plots treated with BioNematon nematicide as control. The BioNematon was prepared by diluting 20 ml of the stock suspension containing 1×10^8 spores/ml in 20 L of distilled water and applied at 40 ml per planting hole at planting and at 40 days after planting to check nematode population on control plots. Initial and final nematode populations were determined for each plot before and after the experiments, respectively. After 90 days, the seedlings were uprooted, and plant growth and disease parameters were evaluated as follows:

3.1 Plant growth parameters evaluated

3.1.1 Shoot height

The height of each plant was taken from the first basal node to the shoot apex using a string, transferred onto a ruler and recorded in centimeters.

3.1.2 Dry weight

The plants were gently uprooted and cut at the first basal node to separate the shoots from roots and dried separately in an oven at 60°C to a constant mass and their weights were recorded in grams.

3.2 RKN disease parameters evaluated

3.2.1 Galling and egg mass indices

Root systems were washed individually and scored for galling indices. Galled roots were stained in phloxine B and scored for egg mass indices. Galling and egg mass indices were scored on a scale of 0–5 where, 0 = no gall or egg masses, 1 = 1–2 galls or egg masses, 2 = 3–10 galls or egg masses, 3 = 11–30 galls or egg masses, 4 = 31–100 galls or egg masses and 5= > 100 galls or egg masses per root system [18, 19].

3.2.2 Endoparasitic nematodes in plant tissues

Another 5 g of the root sample per treatment was stained with Acid Fuchsin for viewing endoparasitic nematodes. The roots were cleared in dilute sodium hypochloride (5.25% NaOCl) for 4 minutes using the sodium-hypochlorite acid fuchsin method described by Byrd et al. [20]. The roots were then rinsed in 100 μm sieve to remove traces of the bleach and stained as described by Hooper et al. [21]. The stained nematodes were enumerated under a stereomicroscope at ×100.

3.2.3 Number of J2s in the soil and roots

Root-knot nematodes were extracted from 200 cm^3 of soil and 5 g of roots using the modified Bearmann extraction tray method as described by Hooper et al. [21]. The roots were cut to 1 cm and blended in 100 ml of water before extraction.

3.2.4 RKN reproduction factor (Rf)

Resistance and susceptibility of tree tomato varieties was based on nematode reproduction factor (Rf) for each variety calculated as a ratio of pf/pi and rated as $Rf \leq 0$ = resistant, $Rf > 0 < 1$ = moderately resistant, $Rf > 1 \geq 5.0$ = tolerant and $Rf > 5.0$ = susceptible [22].

Data on shoot height, dry weights, J2 populations, galling and egg mass indices and nematode Rf were subjected to analysis of variance using SAS software version 9.1. Relationship between galling index (GI) and J2s was determined using regression analysis.

4. Results

4.1 Plant growth parameters in the greenhouse

The shoot heights of inoculated and un-inoculated tree tomato varieties were significantly different ($P \leq 0.05$) from each other, apart from Ruby red. All RKN inoculated varieties recorded lower shoot heights as compared to the control plants (**Table 1** and **Figure 2**).

Treatment	SH(cm)	DSW(g)	DRW(g)
Goldmine+N	38.40 ± 6.64c	6.57 ± 0.93f	2.22 ± 0.99d
Goldmine-N	43.50 ± 5.26a	11.42 ± 1.24d	5.51 ± 2.23b
Ruby red+N	38.68 ± 2.91c	6.49 ± 0.98f	1.47 ± 0.39e
Ruby red-N	38.88 ± 1.53c	7.47 ± 0.80e	1.71 ± 0.65e
Rothamer+N	37.60 ± 2.34d	4.95 ± 1.52 h	1.83 ± 0.70e
Rothamer-N	42.63 ± 4.28b	6.78 ± 0.71f	0.70 ± 0.24f
Red oratia+N	36.75 ± 4.42e	5.71 ± 0.58 g	1.76 ± 0.56e
Red oratia-N	37.45 ± 2.88d	11.02 ± 1.92d	2.19 ± 0.59d
Red L.O + N	33.40 ± 7.51f	16.87 ± 2.41b	12.21 ± 4.89a
Red L.O-N	36.13 ± 3.99e	22.26 ± 2.84a	5.95 ± 1.17b
Grafted+N	28.00 ± 4.02 h	7.56 ± 2.40e	1.82 ± 0.70e
Grafted-N	31.55 ± 2.99 g	12.37 ± 2.49c	3.82 ± 1.58c
P-Value	0.0003	<.0001	0.0025

Means followed by the same letter(s) in the same column are not significantly different ($P \geq 0.05$) according to Tukey's Honestly Significant Difference (HSD). Red L.O = Red light oratia. +N = inoculated with nematodes; -N = un-inoculated treatments.

Table 1.
Effect of root-knot nematodes on mean shoot height (SH), dry shoot weight (DSW) and dry root weight (DRW) of tree tomato varieties in greenhouse experiment (June–September 2019).

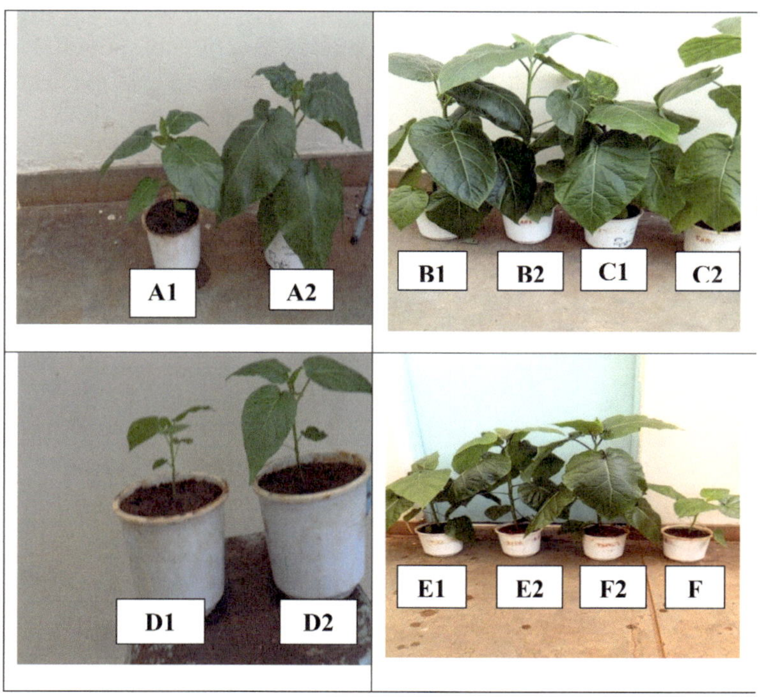

Figure 2.
A1 and A2 = inoculated and un-inoculated red light oratia, B1 and B2 = inoculated and un-inoculated rothamer, C1 and C2 = inoculated and un-inoculated goldmine, D1 and D2 = inoculated and un-inoculated ruby red, E1 and E2 = inoculated and un-inoculated Red oratia and F2 and F1 = uninoculated and inoculated grafted variety in greenhouse experiment. Photos were taken at the end of 90-day period.

The mean dry shoot weight of plants grown on nematode-inoculated soils were lower than that of plants grown on un-inoculated soils for all the tree tomato varieties. There were significant differences ($P \leq 0.05$) between the mean dry shoot weight of plants grown on inoculated and uninoculated soils (**Table 1**).

There were significant differences ($P \leq 0.05$) in the mean dry root weight (DRW) of tree tomato on both inoculated and uninoculated soil. All the tree tomato varieties grown on nematode inoculated soils had their DRW lower than the control treatment except for the cultivar Rothamer and Red light oratia (**Table 1**).

4.2 Root-knot nematode disease parameters in the greenhouse

The mean number of J2s per 5 g of roots was significantly different ($P \leq 0.05$) between varieties except between Ruby red and Red oratia. There were also significant differences ($P \leq 0.05$) in the mean numbers of J2s (pf) per 200 cm^3 of soil in all the tree tomato varieties (**Table 2**).

The mean RKN reproduction factor (Rf) was significantly higher ($P \leq 0.05$) for goldmine compared to other varieties (**Table 2**). Based on the Rf rating, goldmine variety was tolerant (Rf = 4.58) while all the other remaining varieties were moderately resistant in the greenhouse (**Table 2**). A regression analysis revealed a positive significant linear relationship between RKN Rf and nematode gall indices in roots of tree tomato varieties in the greenhouse (**Figure 3**).

The mean galling index for cultivar goldmine was significantly higher ($P \leq 0.05$) compared to other varieties. There was significant difference in the GI between varieties as shown by both untransformed and transformed data in parenthesis (**Table 3**). A regression analysis revealed a positive linear relationship between J2 populations in the roots and nematode gall indices in tree tomato varieties in the greenhouse (**Figure 4**).

There were significant differences ($P \leq 0.05$) in the mean egg mass index (EMI) between varieties while Goldmine, Red light oratia and grafted varieties were not significantly different from each other. The ruby red and red oratia EMI means were the same while Rothamer had the least mean of 2.00 (**Table 3**). The means and P-values of transformed data in parenthesis show significant differences between the EMI means of the varieties.

Treatment	J2s/5 g roots	Pi	Pf	Rf	Host status
Goldmine +N	1042.50 ± 582.50a	2000a	9168.75 ± 51.90a	4.58 ± 0.03a	T
Ruby red +N	253.75 ± 76.25ab	2000a	477.5 ± 202.08de	0.24 ± 0.10d	MR
Rothamer +N	141.25 ± 8.75c	2000a	1546.25 ± 531.57c	0.77 ± 0.27b	MR
Red oratia +N	246.25 ± 21.25ab	2000a	363.75 ± 107.38e	0.18 ± 0.05e	MR
Red light oratia +N	88.75 ± 11.25d	2000a	1785 ± 456.13b	0.89 ± 0.23b	MR
Grafted +N	200.00 ± 5.00b	2000a	651 ± 297.55d	0.33 ± 0.15c	MR
P-Value	0.0018		<.0001	<.0001	

*Means followed by the same letters within the same column are not significantly different ($P \geq 0.05$) with Tukey's test. +N = inoculated with nematodes, Pi = initial nematode populations and Pf = final nematode populations/200 cc of dry soil. **Host status: susceptible (S) when Rf > 5.0, tolerant (T) if 5.0 ≥ Rf > 1, moderately resistant (MR) if 1 > Rf > 0, and resistant (R) [22].*

Table 2.
Mean number of juveniles in soil and roots, Pi, Pf and RKN reproduction factor (Rf) and Tree tomato variety responses to RKNs under greenhouse conditions (June–September 2019).

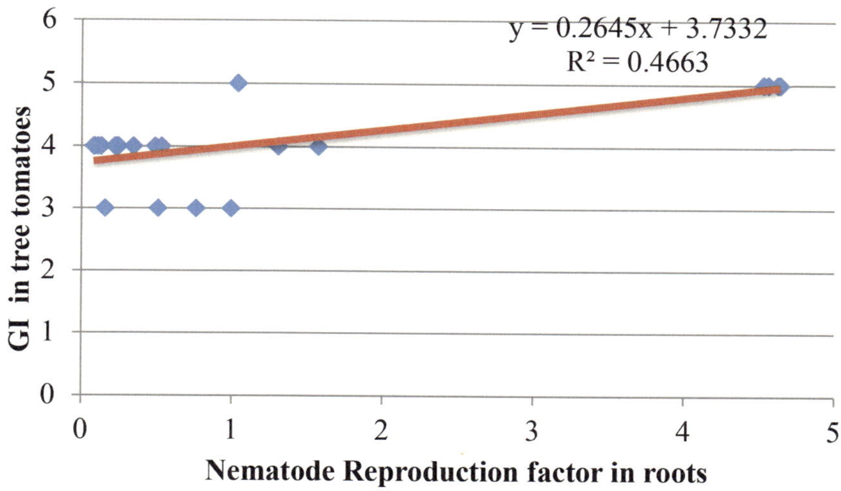

Figure 3.
Relationship between root-knot nematodes reproduction factor and galling index in roots of tree tomatoes in the greenhouse.

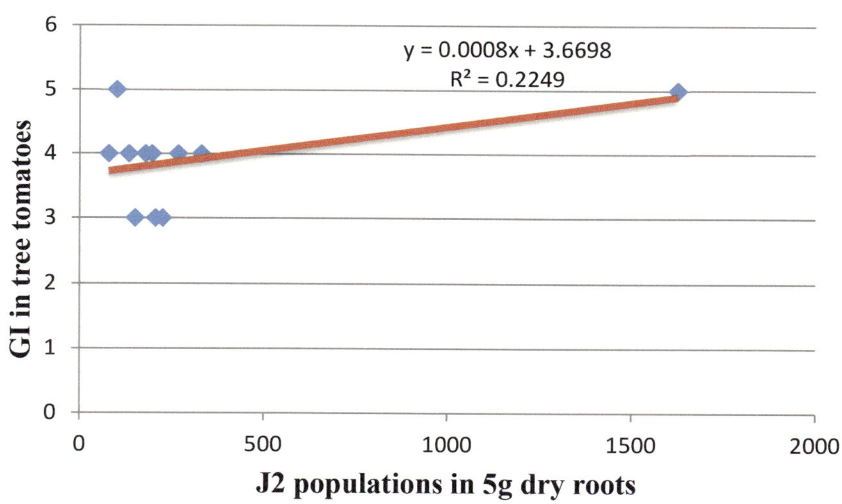

Figure 4.
Relationship between RKN J2 populations and GI in roots of tree tomatoes in the greenhouse.

4.3 Plant growth parameters in the field

The shoot heights were significantly different among the varieties. Goldmine recorded a higher mean shoot height of 29.11 cm in plants grown in nematode-infested soils without BioNematon treatment, followed by Red oratia. Ruby red, Rothamer and Red light oratia had mean heights not significantly different ($P \geq 0.05$) from each other. The Grafted variety grown on nematode-infested plots had the lowest mean height of 21.06 cm (**Table 4**). However, the shoot heights of all tree tomato varieties grown on nematode-infested plots were lower shoot height compared to those on control plots (**Table 4**).

Treatment	GI	EMI
Goldmine+N	5.00 ± 0.00a(0.69a)	4.00 ± 0.00a (0.60a)
Ruby red+N	4.00 ± 0.00ab(0.60ab)	2.50 ± 0.50ab (0.39ab)
Rothamer+N	3.75 ± 0.25b(0.57b)	2.00 ± 0.00b (0.30b)
Red oratia+N	3.75 ± 0.25b(0.57b)	2.50 ± 0.50ab (0.39ab)
Red light oratia+N	4.00 ± 0.41ab(0.59ab)	4.00 ± 0.00a (0.60a)
Grafted+N	3.75 ± 0.25b(0.57b)	4.00 ± 0.00a (0.60a)
P-Value	<.0001(0.0397)	<.0001 (0.0161)

Means followed by the same letters within the same column are not significantly different (P ≥ 0.05) with Tukey's Honestly Significant Difference (HSD). +N = inoculated with nematodes. GI or EMI on a scale of 0–5, where 0 = no galls or egg masses; 1 = 1–2 galls or egg masses; 2 = 3–10 galls or egg masses; 3 = 11–30 galls or egg masses; 4 = 31–100 galls or egg masses and 5= > 100 galls or egg masses per root system [18]. Values in parenthesis are for transformed data.

Table 3.
Mean galling index (GI) and egg mass index (EMI) on Tree tomato varieties under greenhouse conditions (June to September 2019).

Treatment	SH (cm)	DSW (g)	DRW (g)
Goldmine+N	29.11 ± 1.27f	13.07 ± 2.73d	2.89 ± 0.60e
Goldmine+N + BN	44.50 ± 1.43a	20.90 ± 1.41a	5.49 ± 0.45b
Ruby red+N	22.41 ± 1.26 h	7.40 ± 1.72 h	1.92 ± 0.29f
Ruby red+N + BN	30.31 ± 1.21e	8.32 ± 1.49 g	2.44 ± 0.23e
Rothamer+N	22.58 ± 1.33 h	9.44 ± 2.17f	2.14 ± 0.64e
Rothamer+N + BN	32.57 ± 1.00d	13.07 ± 1.80d	3.18 ± 0.52d
Red oratia+N	26.06 ± 1.12 g	16.20 ± 4.01b	4.60 ± 1.25c
Red oratia +N + BN	39.38 ± 1.10b	20.66 ± 2.84a	6.23 ± 1.37a
Red light oratia+N	22.13 ± 1.15 h	9.82 ± 2.26f	2.55 ± 0.56e
Red light oratia+N + BN	37.09 ± 0.95c	14.57 ± 0.92c	4.36 ± 0.75c
Grafted+N	21.06 ± 0.72i	9.01 ± 1.19f	3.02 ± 0.52d
Grafte +N + BN	29.64 ± 0.96f	12.32 ± 0.89e	3.43 ± 0.62d
P-Value	<.0001	<.0001	0.0004

+N = nematode-infested soil; BN = BioNematon (nematicide). Means followed by the same letters within the same column are not significantly different (P ≥ 0.05) according to Tukey's Honestly Significant Difference (HSD).

Table 4.
Effect of root-knot nematodes on mean shoot height (SH), dry shoot weight (DSW) and dry root weight (DRW) of tree tomato varieties in field experiment (June to August 2019).

The dry shoot weights of all the varieties on nematode-infested plots were significantly different (P ≤ 0.05) as compared to those on control plots. The dry shoot weights of plants on control plots were higher than those on nematode-infested plots without BioNematon treatment. Red oratia variety recorded a mean dry shoot weight of 16.20 g followed by Goldmine and Red light oratia on nematode-infested plots. Ruby red recorded the lowest mean dry shoot weight of 7.40 g (**Table 4**).

The mean dry root weight of the tree tomato varieties differed significantly (P ≤ 0.05) from each other between plants on nematode-infested plots as compared to those on control plots, except the grafted variety. The dry root weight of plants on nematode-infested plots without BioNematon were lower than that of the controls (**Table 4**). Red oratia recorded the highest mean of 4.60 g followed by Grafted and Goldmine varieties (3.02 g and 2.89 g, respectively) on nematode-infested plots. Ruby red had the lowest mean dry root weight of 1.92 g (**Table 4**).

4.4 Root-knot nematode disease parameters in the field

The number of J2s in 5 g of roots was significantly different ($P \leq 0.05$) between tree tomato varieties. The grafted variety and red light oratia had the highest mean number of J2 populations in the roots with 388.33 J2s/5 g and 294.20 J2s/5 g of roots, respectively. Red oratia had the lowest mean number of J2s for plants grown on nematode-infested plots without BioNematon treatment (**Table 5**). The number of J2s in 5 g of roots for plants grown on control plots had a lower number of nematodes as compared to those on untreated plots.

There were significant differences ($P \leq 0.05$) between the mean numbers of J2s in the rhizosphere soils of the tree tomato varieties. The Grafted variety recorded a mean of 80.00 J2s (pf), followed by Goldmine variety with a mean of 61.67 J2s and Red light oratia with a mean of 46.67 J2s per 200 cm^3 of soil (**Table 5**).

The mean RKN Rf was significantly different ($P \leq 0.05$) among the varieties with goldmine having the highest mean Rf of 5.78. The Grafted variety had a mean Rf of 4.26 followed by Red light oratia with 4.07 (**Table 5**). Plants on nematode-infested plots without BioNematon treatment were rated for susceptibility or resistance to RKNs [22]. Goldmine (Rf = 5.78) was rated as susceptible (S),

Treatment	J2s/5 g dry roots	Pi	Pf	Rf	Host status
Goldmine + N	53.30 ± 35.83c	10.00 ± 2.88 h	61.67 ± 22.19b	5.78 ± 1.30a	S
Goldmine + N + BN	7.00 ± 0.1.4 g	9.17 ± 2.22i	8.09 ± 2.00 g	0.62 ± 0.04e	—
Ruby red+N	21.70 ± 4.17d	18.33 ± 8.82d	17.50 ± 5.77f	1.60 ± 0.96c	MR
Ruby red + N + BN	6.89 ± 0.20 g	16.17 ± 4.67e	10.00 ± 1.90 g	0.44 ± 0.07e	—
Rothamer + N	15.83 ± 0.83e	19.17 ± 4.64c	19.17 ± 2.21e	1.10 ± 0.21d	MR
Rothamer + N + BN	6.23 ± 0.10 g	18.50 ± 1.76d	10.12 ± 3.03 g	0.35 ± 0.50e	—
Red oratia + N	12.50 ± 1.44f	6.67 ± 3.01j	25.83 ± 7.12d	1.50 ± 0.14c	MR
Red oratia +N + BN	7.50 ± 1.1 g	18.17 ± 1.88d	10.94 ± 2.97 g	0.47 ± 0.06e	—
Red L.O + N	294.20 ± 187.14b	13.33 ± 2.21f	46.67 ± 15.43c	4.07 ± 1.73b	T
Red L.O + N + BN	6.86 ± 1.00 g	43.67 ± 33.21a	11.82 ± 3.40 g	0.21 ± 0.09e	—
Grafted + N	388.33 ± 87.61a	27.5 ± 15.00b	80 ± 11.27a	4.26 ± 1.24b	T
Grafted +N + BN	6.39 ± 0.10 g	12.73 ± 2.39 g	8.42 ± 1.05 g	0.48 ± 0.08e	—
P-Value	0.0007	0.0041	<.0001	<.0001	

Means followed by the same letters along the same column are not significantly different ($P \geq 0.05$) according to Tukey's Honestly Significant Difference (HSD). +N = nematode infested plots; +BN=Plots treated with BioNematon (nematicide); Red L.O = Red light oratia. Pi = initial nematode population per 200 cm^3 of soil, Pf = final nematode population per 200 cm^3 of soil. Rf is based on Pf/Pi rated on a scale of 0–5. Host status (susceptible or resistant); susceptible when $Rf > 5.0$, tolerant if $5.0 \geq Rf > 1$, moderately resistant if $1 > Rf > 0$, and resistant when $Rf \leq 0$) [22].

Table 5.
Mean number of juveniles in soil and roots and RKN reproduction factor (Rf) on tree tomato varieties under field conditions.

Treatment	GI	EMI
Goldmine+N	3.38 ± 0.20a (0.58a)	4.67 ± 0.33a (0.67a)
Goldmine+ N + BN	0.32 ± 0.15e (0.20e)	0.90 ± 2.17e (0.07e)
Ruby red+N	0.75 ± 0.15c (0.05c)	1.33 ± 0.33d (0.10d)
Ruby red+ N + BN	0.30 ± 0.18e (0.01e)	0.44 ± 0.09e (0.03e)
Rothamer+N	0.38 ± 0.16d (0.03d)	1.33 ± 0.33d (0.10d)
Rothamer+ N + BN	0.33 ± 0.10 e(0.19e)	0.50 ± 0.07e (0.03e)
Red oratia+N	0.79 ± 0.20c (0.06c)	2.33 ± 0.33c (0.36c)
Red oratia+ N + BN	0.29 ± 0.14e (0.13e)	0.21 ± 0.69e (0.02e)
Red light oratia+N	2.00 ± 0.26b (0.27b)	3.00 ± 0.58b (0.46b)
Red L.O+ N + BN	0.25 ± 0.11e (0.15e)	0.75 ± 0.07e (0.04e)
Grafted+N	3.79 ± 0.19a (0.56a)	4.67 ± 0.33a (0.67a)
Grafted+ N + BN	0.31 ± 0.21e (0.26e)	1.02 ± 3.00e (0.08e)
P-Value	<.0001 (<.0001)	<.0001(<0.0001)

Means followed by the same letter(s) along the same column are not significantly different ($P \geq 0.05$) according to Tukey's Honestly Significant Difference (HSD) test. Means in parenthesis are for log-transformed data. +N = nematode infested plots; +BN=Plots-treated with BioNematon (nematicide); Red L.O = Red light oratia. GI or EMI on a scale of 0–5, where 0 = no galls or egg masses; 1 = 1–2 galls or egg masses; 2 = 3–10 galls or egg masses; 3 = 11–30 galls or egg masses; 4 = 31–100 galls or egg masses and 5= > 100 galls or egg masses per root system [18]. Values in parenthesis are for transformed data.

Table 6.
Mean galling index (GI) and egg mass index (EMI) on tree tomato varieties under field conditions.

Grafted (Rf = 4.26) and Red light oratia (Rf = 4.07) were tolerant (T). Ruby red, Rothamer and Red oratia (Rf = 1.60, 1.10 and 1.50, respectively) were moderately resistant (MR) (**Table 5**).

The mean galling indices differed significantly ($P \leq 0.05$) between the varieties (**Table 6**). The grafted and goldmine varieties had the highest GI followed by red light oratia. All the plants on nematode-infested plots without BioNematon treatments had significantly higher mean number of GI as compared to those on control plots (**Table 6**).

The mean EMI indices differed significantly ($P \leq 0.05$) among the varieties except between ruby red and rothamer on nematode-infested plots without BioNematon treatment (**Table 6**). Goldmine and grafted varieties had the highest mean EMI (**Table 6**).

5. Discussion

There were significant differences in the responses of tree tomato varieties to RKNs in the greenhouse test and also in the field. The shoot heights of all tree tomato varieties differed significantly both in the greenhouse and in the field. However, plants in the greenhouse had higher shoot heights than those in the field. A conducive and ambient environment in the greenhouse could be the reason for this observation. This could also be due to harsh environmental conditions and the interaction of the tree tomato with mixed nematode populations in the field. The dry shoot weight and dry root weight of tree tomato varieties varied significantly in both greenhouse and field tests. Tree tomatoes on RKN-infested soils were lighter and shorter compared to the control in both experiments. This could be due to nematode damage to the root system, which interferes with water and mineral uptake.

The variety response to RKNs ranged between tolerant for goldmine and moderately resistant for ruby red, rothamer, red oratia, red light oratia and grafted varieties in the greenhouse. Ruby red, rothamer and red oratia were consistently moderately resistant in both greenhouse and field tests. Red light oratia and grafted varieties were both moderately resistant in the greenhouse and tolerant in the field. Goldmine was tolerant in the greenhouse and susceptible in the field. Change of responses from tolerant to susceptible for goldmine could be due to mixed nematode populations, varied nematode pathotypes and variations in population density in the greenhouse and field. These could have also been the reasons for loss of moderate resistance to tolerance in red light oratia and grafted varieties between greenhouse and field tests. Maleita [23] reported that moderately resistant and tolerant varieties can become susceptible when the RKN population and environmental conditions vary. The Goldmine variety was found to harbor comparatively high numbers of J2s, high egg mass and gall indices in both greenhouse and field tests. In addition, red light oratia and grafted varieties recorded high galling and egg mass indices. However, the moderately resistant varieties had comparatively lower nematode reproduction factors. These varieties could have resistant genes [24].

The moderately resistant varieties should be promoted to farmers through extension programs so as to avoid losses that come as a result of planting susceptible varieties. These varieties can also be used in breeding and seed certification programs for quality production of tree tomato yields through improved phytosanitation of planting materials.

Moderately resistant varieties can be used in integrated pest management strategies since they could have a resistant gene (Mi gene). Resistance to RKN invasion may trigger the plant to form necrotic cells at the point of infection to stop J2 development. However, very high genetic variability of RKNs has brought about the occurrence of virulent races that can reproduce in plants carrying the resistant genes. These are pathotypes that break resistance [24–26]. The information on tree tomato variety responses to RKNs can be helpful to farmers in selecting the varieties to plant on RKN-infested farms.

The plants in the Solanaceae family are susceptible to RKN infection and other PPNs, hence, supporting higher nematode populations [27, 28]. The root-knot nematodes were found to be associated with all six screened tree tomato varieties in both tests. Studies on indigenous leafy vegetables by Nchore et al. [29] and Wangai et al. [28] on coffee germplasms reported variations in responses to RKN similar to these findings. Another study on sweet potatoes reported that susceptibility to RKN could be due to the presence of unfavorable alleles that reduce resistance [30]. Failure of the infective J2s to penetrate, form feeding sites, mature and reproduce in the plant roots may have been the cause of the observed moderate resistance [29–31]. The observed differences in responses of tree tomato varieties to RKNs could also be due to genetic variations between themselves, and this explains the differences in galling index, egg mass index and nematode reproduction factor [24].

All tree tomato varieties on nematode-inoculated/infested soils had lower plant growth parameters. The stunting and yellowing of leaves observed on susceptible plants was due to RKN damage on the roots that interfered with water and mineral uptake. Stunting is caused by the redirection of manufactured food to nematode feeding sites [32–34].

6. Conclusion

Ruby red, rothamer and red oratia varieties were moderately resistant while red light oratia and grafted varieties were tolerant and goldmine was susceptible to RKNs.

7. Recommendations

i. The identified moderately resistant varieties (ruby red, rothamer and red oratia) and tolerant varieties (red light oratia and grafted) should be promoted to farmers to manage RKNs in tree tomato through rotational programs.

ii. Moderately resistant and tolerant varieties should be incorporated into breeding programs to manage RKNs in tree tomato.

iii. Further research is needed to characterize the RKN species infecting tree tomato.

Author details

Waswa Stanlous Juma[1,2*], Waceke Joyce Wajohi[2] and Nchore Shem Bonuke[3]

1 Department of Biological and Environmental Sciences, Kibabii University, Bungoma, Kenya

2 Department of Agricultural Science and Technology, Kenyatta University, Kenya

3 Department of Plant Sciences, Kenyatta University, Nairobi, Kenya

*Address all correspondence to: waswastanlous@yahoo.com

References

[1] Ramirez F, Grijalra R, Navarrete X, Guerrero R. Phytoparasitic Nematodes Associated with Tree Tomato (*Solanum betaceum* Cav.) in the Provinces of Imbura, Pichincha and Tungurahua, Ecuador. Interoceanic Km 14 1/2. Tumbaco, Ecuador: The MAGAP Farm; 2015

[2] Ramírez-Gil JG, Gil-Aguirre A, Morales-Osorio JG. Etiología de enfermedades del cultivo de tomate de árbol (*Solanum betaceum* CAV.). Revista de Protección Vegetal. 2017;**32**(1):33-51

[3] United States Agency on International Development, Agriculture Fisheries and Food Authority of Kenya. Horticulture Validated Report. 2014. pp. 51-52. Available from: www.agricultureauthority.go.ke/Horticulture-Validated-Report.2014

[4] Reddy PP. Impact of climate change on insect pests, pathogens and nematodes. Pest Management sin Horticultural Ecosystems. 2013;**19**(2):225-233

[5] Agarwal S, Rao AV. Tomato lycopene and its role in human health and chronic diseases. CMAJ: Canadian Medical Association Journal = Journal de l'Association medicale canadienne. 2000;**163**(6):739-744

[6] Waswa SJ, Waceke JW, Nchore SB. Occurrence and abundance of phytonematodes in tree tomato (*Solanum betaceum* Cav.) farming systems in Kenya. Journal of Agriculture. 2020;7(7):1-10. Available from: http://www.researchjournali.com/pdf.5605.pdf

[7] Coyne DL, Cortada L, Dalzell JJ, Claudius-Cole AO, Haukeland S, Luambano N, et al. Plant-parasitic nematodes and food security in sub-Saharan Africa. Annual Review of Phytopathology. 2018;**56**:381-403

[8] Jones JT, Haegeman A, Danchin EGJ, Gaur HS, Helder J, Jones MGK, et al. Top 10 plant-parasitic nematodes in molecular plant pathology. Molecular Plant Pathology. 2013;**14**:946-961

[9] Vásquez PU, Soria CA. Nematodos parásitos asociados con tomate de árbol (*Solanum betaceum* Cav.) en la sierra del Ecuador. Revista Ecuatoriana de Medicina y Ciencias Biológicas. 2017;**38**(2):107-118

[10] Oxfarm. 2017. Available from: http://www.oxfarmorganic.com/our-products/tree-tomato/tips-on-how-to-get-over-20kgs-tree-from-tree-tomato-farming/

[11] Prohens J, Nuez F. The Tamarillo (Cyphomandra betacea) a review of a promising small fruit crop. Small Fruits Review. 2001;**1**(2):43-68

[12] Muriithi C, Matiri F, Kihanda F, Maina D, Kasungo F. Evaluation of potential of tree tomato production and marketing in Eastern Kenya for improved nutrition and food security. In: Joint Proceedings of the 27th Soil Science Society of East Africa and the 6th African Soil Science Society Conference; 20-25 October 2023

[13] Korayem AM, Youssef MMA, Mohamed MMM, Lashein AMS. A survey of plant parasitic nematodes associated with different plants in North Sinai. Middle East J Agriculture Research. 2014;**3**(3):522-529

[14] Oxfarm. 2019. Available from: www.oxfarm.com/our-products/tree-tomato/tree-tomato-farming-made-easy-in-Kenya

[15] Rahman SSA, Zain SM, Mat MB, Sidam AK, Othman RY, Mohamed Z. Population distribution of plant-parasitic nematodes of bananas in peninsular Malaysia. Sains Malaysiana. 2014;**43**(2):175-183

[16] Agriculture and Food Authority, Government of Kenya and Kenya National Bureau of Statistics. 2015-2016. p. 41. Available from: www.agricultureauthority.go.ke/Horticulture-Validated-Report.2015-2016

[17] Hussey RS, Barker KR. A comparison of methods of collecting inocula of *Meloidogyne* species including a new technique. Plant Disease Report. 1973;**57**:1025e1028

[18] Quesenberry KH, Baltensperger DD, Dunn RA, Wilcox CJ, Hardy SR. Selection for tolerance to root-knot nematodes in red clover. Crop Science. 1989;**29**:62-66

[19] Taylor AL, Sasser JN. Biology, Identification and Control of Root-Knot Nematodes (*Meloidogyne* Species). North Carolina State University Graphics; 1978. pp. 1-111

[20] Byrd DW, Kirkpatrick T, Baker R. An improved technique for clearing and staining plant tissue for detection of nematodes. Journal of Nematology. 1983;**15**:142-143

[21] Hooper DJ, Hallmann J, Subbotin SA. Methods for extraction, processing and detection of and soil nematodes. In: Luc M, Sikora R, Bridge A, editors. Plant Parasitic Nematodes in Subtropical and Tropical Agriculture. 2nd ed. Wallingford, UK: CAB International; 2005. pp. 53-86. Available from: https://www.crfg.org/pubs/ff/tamarillo.html

[22] Zhang F, Schmitt DP. Host status of 32 plant species to *Meloidogyne konaensis*. Journal of Nematology. 1994;**26**(4S):744

[23] Maleta CM. Biology and Ecology of the Root-Knot Nematodes *Meloidogyne Hispanica*: A Species of Emerging Importance [PhD thesis]. Portugal: University of Coimbra; 2011

[24] Singh SK, Khurma UR. Susceptibility of six tomato cultivars to the root-knot nematode, *Meloidogyne incognita*. The South Pacific Journal of Natural and Applied Sciences. 2007;**25**(1):73-77

[25] Castagnone-Sereno P. Genetic variability and adaptive evolution in parthenogenetic root-knot nematodes. Heredity. 2006;**96**(4):282

[26] Jacquet M, Bongiovanni M, Martinez M, Verschave P, Wajnberg E, Castagnone-Sereno P. Variation in resistance to the root-knot nematode *Meloidogyne incognita* in tomato genotypes bearing the mi gene. Plant Pathology. 2005;**54**(2):93-99

[27] Nchore SB. Incidence, Prevalence and Management of Root-Knot Nematodes *(Meloidogyne Spp.)* on Selected Indigenous Leafy Vegetables in Kisii and Trans-Mara Counties, Kenya [Msc thesis]. Nairobi, Kenya: Kenyatta University; 2012

[28] Wangai KJ, Nzesya MJ, Maina MW, Peter WM, Elijah GK. Reaction of selected coffee germplasm to root-knot nematodes in Kenya. Journal of Natural Sciences Research. 2014;**4**(3):68-75

[29] Nchore SB, Waceke JW, Kariuki GM. Efficacy of selected agroindustrial wastes in managing root-knot nematodes on black nightshade in Kenya. ISRN Agronomy. 2012:2012

[30] Karuri HW, Olago D, Neilson R, Mararo E, Villinger J. A survey of root knot nematodes and resistance to *Meloidogyne incognita* in sweet potato

varieties from Kenyan fields. Crop Protection. 2017;**92**:114-121

[31] Sujatha R, Vethamoni PI, Manivannan N, Sivakumar M. Screening of tomato genotypes for root knot nematode (*Meloidogyne incognita* Kofoid and white chit wood). International Journal of Current Microbiology and Applied Sciences. 2017;**6**(3):1525-1533

[32] Hunt DJ, Palomares-Rius JE, Manzanilla-López RH. Identification, morphology and biology of plant parasitic nematodes. Plant Parasitic Nematodes in Subtropical and Tropical Agriculture. 2018;**20**:20-61

[33] Wallace HR. Interactions between nematodes and other factors on plants. Journal of Nematology. 1983;**15**(2):221

[34] Jaiteh F. Screening tomato (*Solanum lycopersicum* L.) genotypes for resistance to root-knot nematodes (*Meloidogyne* species) [M.sc thesis]. Kumasi, Ghana: Kwame Nguruma University of Science and Technology; 2010